The World's Most Convenient Diet

The World's Most Convenient Diet

By Zoe Ann Komaransky, R.D.
Linda Lackney, R.D.

Published by
Turnbull & Willoughby
1151 West Webster Avenue
Chicago, Illinois 60614

Text copyright © 1984 by Linda Lackney, RD. & Zoe Ann Komaransky, RD. Manufactured in the United States of America. First Printing November, 1984

All rights reserved. No part of this book may be used or reproduced in any manner whatsoever without written permission except in the case of reviews.
ISBN 0-943084-10-5
5 4 3 2 1

Cover and book design by Michael Brierton

ATTENTION: Turnbull & Willoughby books are available at quantity discounts with bulk purchase for educational, business or sales promotional use. For information, please write to: Bulk Sales Department, Turnbull & Willoughby, 1151 W. Webster, Chicago, IL., 60614.

Every effort has been made to contact the copyright and trademark owners or their representatives for correct representation of their products. If there have been any omissions, please notify us and we will rectify them in future printings.

The World's Most Convenient Diet

**To our families and Clarence Birdseye
with
a special acknowledgement to Mary Pat**

The World's Most Convenient Diet

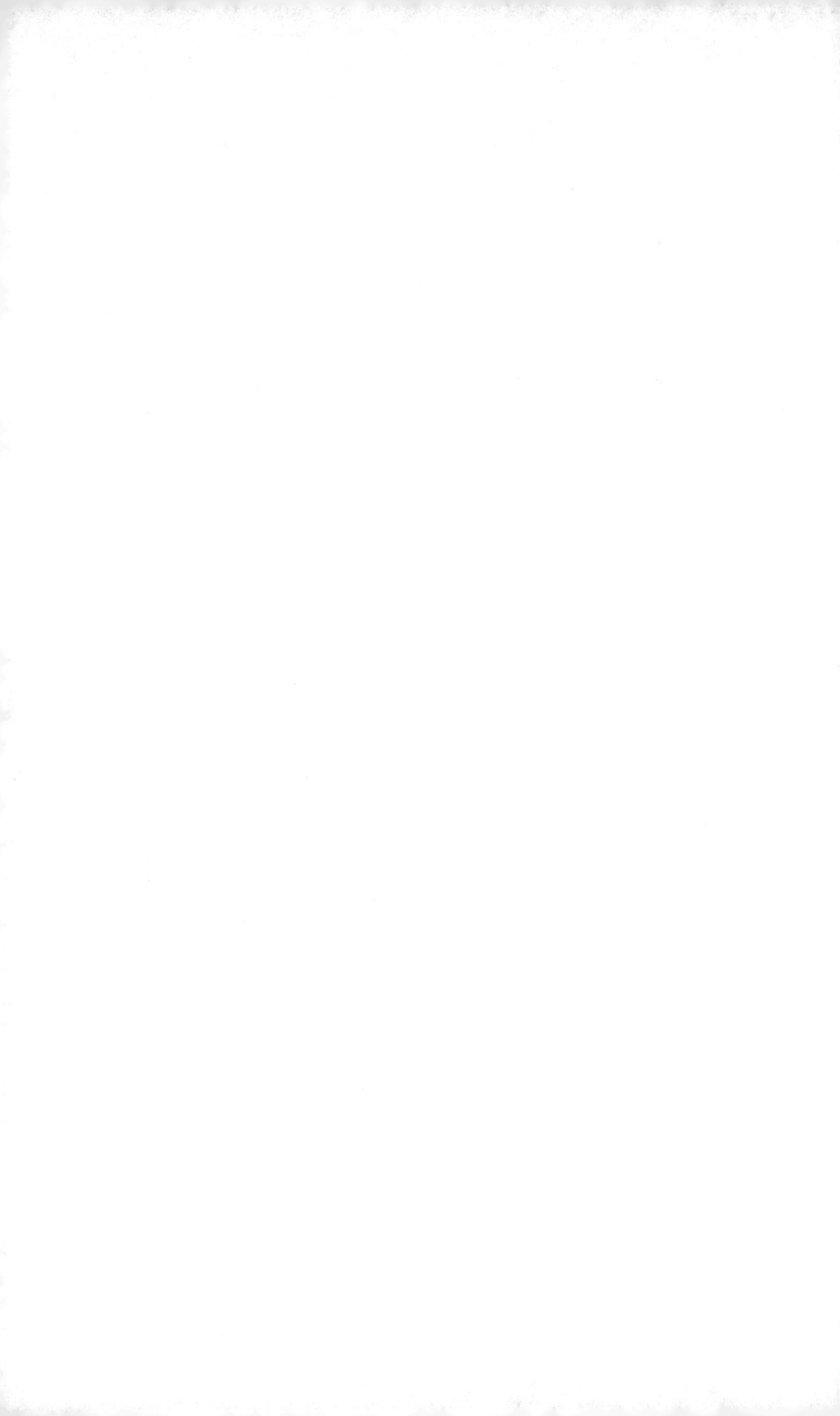

Contents

	Introduction	1
1	The Easy Weigh Off	1
2	The Convenience Quotient	7

    9 Finding Your CQ
    9 Convenience Quotient Quiz
  10 Scoring
  10 Discussion

3	And Now The World's Most Convenient Diet	13

  15 Basic Directions
  19 Fresh Fruit Stand
  21 Super Salad Bar
  22 Free Foods

4	Seven-Day Sample Plan	25

  27 Shopping Guide For The First Week
  29 One-Week Sample Menu

5	The Menu Planner	35

Breakfast

  39 Ready-to-Eat Cereals
  49 Hot Cereals
  51 Toaster Breakfasts
  53 Bakery Breakfasts
  56 Miscellaneous Breakfasts

Lunch

  61 Fast Food Fare
  62 Simple Sandwiches
  66 Hot and Hearty
  79 When You're the Cook

Dinner

  83 Fast Food
  84 Heat and Eat
  93 Cool and Quick
  94 Home Cooking

continued

6	Recommended Multivitamin-With-Minerals Supplements	**97**
7	**Taking You Through Thick To Thin**	**101**
	103 Determining a Target Weight	
	104 Developing a New Approach to Eating	
	105 Seven Techniques to Alter Your Eating Habits	
	106 Your Eating Signals: What Are They?	
	107 Fitness vs. Fat	
8	**Nutrients**	**109**
	111 Protein	
	112 Fat	
	113 Carbohydrates	
	114 Fluids and Electrolytes	
	114 Fiber	
	115 Vitamins and Minerals	
9	**Supermarket Savvy**	**119**
	121 The Produce Department	
	134 Stocking the Cupboard	
	133 The Refrigerator and Freezer Sections	
10	**Diet Dialogue**	**137**
11	**Thin Conclusions**	**153**
	The Menu-Planner Index	**157**
	Manufacturers' Index	**171**
	References	**185**
	Authors' Biographies	**199**

Introduction

Introduction

What do the words "convenience foods" suggest to you? Wide selection, right? Little or no preparation. Delicious taste.

How about the word "diet"? Most images associated with dieting are negative: boredom, drudgery, complicated formulas. The only good part about dieting, it seems, is the weight loss. And all too often, even that's temporary.

Now it's time to blend the necessity of dieting with the modern joy of convenience foods. The result is a program that features the best of both worlds – a diet that's effective in trimming off excess weight, but which is also fun and easy. It's a diet that's so convenient you won't find yourself abandoning it after two weeks and going back to your self-defeating eating habits. It's a plan that's professionally designed to provide good nutrition without sacrificing taste.

It is, in sum, *The World's Most Convenient Diet*. If you're interested in slimming down but still enjoying pizza, tacos, hamburgers and those delicious new frozen gourmet meals, this diet's for you.

A convenience food is any product that's ready to eat or almost completely prepared in advance for the consumer. Breakfast cereals, condensed soups and fast foods are all part of the industry. And what an industry it is! The Stouffers Food Corporation alone had revenues of $133 million in 1974, and its steadily escalating sales are expected to top $1 billion in 1985.

What sparked this explosion? The microwave oven is only a minor factor. As registered dietitians who have counseled thousands of dieters, we're aware that the country's changing lifestyles and eating habits are contributing to the soaring popularity of convenience foods. Households are smaller and more hectic. More than half of the married women work outside the home and nearly half of the husbands help with grocery shopping. Single people are busy with their jobs and social activities. Complicated and time-consuming diets just don't fit in with today's fast pace. Even those who love to cook may be able to pursue that activity only as a hobby during their free time instead of as part of their daily routine.

As demand for convenience foods has increased, the marketplace has responded with better and more varied products. Frozen dinners no longer carry the stigma of tasting worse than their cardboard cartons. Many are delicious and some are available in such elegant combinations that a recent advertising campaign promoted their use for fine dining with vintage wine aboard a yacht!

Technological advances can be credited with boosting the quality of convenience foods. Clarence Birdseye, who introduced frozen peas, realized that freezing food was an excellent way to preserve nutrients and taste. If proper preparation, freezing and packaging procedures are used, vitamin and mineral losses are minimal whether the items are fruits, vegetables or meats. Over the years, new ways of heating foods more efficiently and then freezing them more rapidly have been developed, ensuring quality as close to fresh as possible. The quality often can be considered better than fresh because enzymes or organisms that can cause spoilage are destroyed or inhibited in the food processing.

Innovations in packaging also have contributed to the higher quality of convenience foods. The better the package, the better the food holds up under storage. Vacuum-sealed pouches and tightly wrapped plates with additional covers are common on today's market. And with the smaller portion sizes now available, reheating times are shorter, meaning improved retention of flavor and nutrients.

With convenience foods enjoying unprecedented popularity, it's about time they were incorporated into a sensible weight-loss plan. A good diet uses appealing foods that can be eaten during the reducing period as well as during the long term. And any worthwhile weight-reduction plan will make it as easy as possible for the dieter to stick with his or her resolve to lose weight.

Some might be surprised to see "fast foods" included on our diet. But too many people throw all fast foods into the so-called "junk-food" category, even though there's a major difference between the nutritional value of various fast foods. For instance, both pizza and soda pop are typically labeled "junk foods," yet these foods have little in common other than providing a source of calories. It is possible for pizza to contain vitamins, minerals and protein in such appropriate levels that it can be included in a sensible weight loss plan.

Our diet is the result of carefully selecting foods based on their nutritional content. We didn't focus our attention solely on calories. Protein, fat, sodium, vitamins and minerals were also important considerations. Some fast-food combinations, for instance, can lack vitamins A and C, and yet contain substantial amounts of high-quality protein. So we have combined such foods with a variety of fruits and vegetables to ensure adequate vitamins as well as protein.

In other words, we have done all the nutritional research for you. Entree per entree, product per product, calories and nutrients do vary, but you will always be within safe nutritional limits by sticking to our predetermined diet plan. Any combination of menus assures protein in amounts meeting or exceeding the standards set by the National Research Council's Board of Food and Nutrition. The calorie content for women will average 1,200 calories per day, and for men, 1,500 calories. The sodium will generally range from 2,000 to 3,500 milligrams, a safe level for healthy individuals. Fat levels are held at 35 percent or less. This is below the typical 40 percent found in many American diets. If desired, the dieter can control cholesterol amounts by choosing vegetable margarine, skim milk and meals that do not have eggs as an entree.

We eliminated some otherwise suitable foods from our plan because of such factors as sodium and fat content. For instance, sometimes the total number of calories in a diet plan looks correct, but too many of the calories may come from fat. That makes it difficult to get enough protein and carbohydrates into the diet. As for sodium, there appears to be a trend among manufacturers toward a gradual reduction in sodium. While research into the connection between sodium and health is continuing, it appears prudent to decrease the average sodium intake when possible.

Our diet isn't an endorsement of any specific products. Rather, it's a listing of foods that meet our nutritional criteria. We were able to select foods only from those companies that provided us with their product information. This doesn't mean that products missing from the list would necessarily prove unacceptable for this or any other healthy eating plan.

And finally, please check with your physician before starting *any* diet, including our program. It should be determined whether any special therapeutic modifications are necessary.

As professional dietitians, we've seen how many people fail to adhere to their diets because the methods used are time-consuming, complicated, boring or – worst of all – dangerous. We think it's time that a diet should be safe, effective *and* convenient. This is it. Go ahead – enjoy yourself and lose weight at the same time!

Chapter One
The Easy Weigh Off

The Easy Weigh Off

"What goes up must come down" applies to gravity, but not your weight. You may have found that the well-known corollary – "the bigger they are, the harder they fall" – better reflects your struggles to reduce.

When it comes to dieting, we're all looking for the "easy weigh off." It's so simple to put pounds on that it seems only fair they should come off easily. It would be great if weight reduction did not demand low-calorie foods, lots of measuring or monotony. Just the time necessary for preparing diet meals is at a premium for most of us. What about those fantastic, already prepared foods everyone is putting in their grocery carts? Somehow it seems a dieter should be able to eat a *Stouffer's®* French Bread Pizza and still lose weight.

We agree. For most of us, the concept of convenience is a high priority in just about anything we do, including dieting. Too many diets have been abandoned because the demand for time becomes an obstacle. Diets must offer variety. Some foods wear thin long before we do! Anyone who has tried a "tunnel-vision" plan knows this. Two weeks of fruit and cottage cheese or a liquid supplement makes the switch to regular food an occasion to binge.

The question becomes obvious: Can convenience foods be used on a weight-loss diet? We feel they certainly can be. The key is knowing how to select them. That is why we created *The World's Most Convenient Diet*. In our work as registered dietitians*, we know there are literally hundreds of products that can be used to make dieting much easier, much better tasting and more interesting. We have surveyed the most recent nutrient information available from brand-name manufacturers to determine which items can be used and still allow a person to lose weight.

Our product selection task began with setting nutritional criteria. In this way, we could allow for the variance between items and yet meet a predetermined daily nutrient average. The day's total calories approximate 1,200 for women and 1,500 for men. Minimum daily protein requirements are 45 and 60 grams respectively for females and males. The calorie and protein levels were set to ensure the dieter received adequate amounts of these important nutrients.

Two other nutritional criteria, fat and sodium, were important in our selection process. These two nutrients had to be limited to make sure the dieter would not get excessive amounts. Fat was limited to approximately 35 percent or less of the day's calories. Sodium limits were set to keep the average daily intake at 3,500 milligrams or less.

---

*The title, registered dietitian, signified by the initials R.D. following the professional's name, indicates the person has met specific requirements in nutrition, food management and clinical dietetics. Meeting these requirements means the dietitian has earned a college degree in a nutrition-related field. Clinical experience is either integrated into the four-year college program or incorporated in an internship following graduation. The candidate must pass the national registration examination to become registered. Seventy-five hours of continuing education need to be accumulated every five years to maintain the title.

To the entrees chosen by this process, we added fresh fruits, vegetables and the option of whole grain breads. Not only does this help keep the diet balanced, but it also addresses the concern of including fiber in the daily menu. Low-fat milk and margarine round out many of the meals. We have compiled a list of vitamin-with-minerals supplements that meet, but do not "over exceed," Recommended Daily Allowance levels.

Technically, you've been shown how *The World's Most Convenient Diet* was conceived. How does it work for you? Very simply, now that all the investigative work has been done. The diet begins with a seven-day planned menu that you may follow for the first week of your weight-loss program. This is to acquaint you with the variety of foods that can be achieved with just a little imagination. A shopping list for the first week is included to make dieting even more convenient. You choose your fruit from our Fresh Fruit Stand and build your salads at our Super Salad Bar.

Following the sample first week program you will find more than 300 meals with which to plan your daily menu. Items have been grouped to accommodate your lifestyle. For example, some lunches are listed in a simple sandwich category for those who brown-bag it. There is a hot and hearty lunch section for those who are at home or have access to a microwave oven at work. Fast foods also are an option. Each day you choose one breakfast, one lunch and one dinner. Following this rule, you will always remain within predetermined nutrient limits. The potential combinations are endless and all equally simple. You can repeat your favorites but we recommend varying your selections.

Versatility was taken one step further in *The World's Most Convenient Diet*. We know everyone has the urge to get out the cookbooks and dirty some pots and pans once in a while. For those days, we have included guidelines for non-convenience meals. These guidelines indicate proper serving sizes for meats, breads, vegetables, fruit and fat selections. This way you will have the option of preparing meals from scratch while still adhering to the diet plan.

The weight loss that can be expected on this diet will vary with each individual. The total amount of pounds you need to lose and the amount of exercise you get daily will affect the weight-loss rate. Our experience with participants shows an initial weight loss of three to five pounds the first week and an average loss of two pounds per week thereafter. This can add up to a 9 to 11 pound weight loss in four weeks. You do not have to switch back to normal food at the end of the diet because you never switched to diet food. When you have reached your target weight, you may use *The World's Most Convenient Diet* two or three days a week to help maintain your weight. The diet is well balanced and can be followed as needed.

In addition to the menu planning guide, you will find this book contains other valuable information needed to achieve successful weight loss. In our "Thick to Thin" chapter, you'll learn how to determine an ideal body weight and then change your approach to eating. We've included a "Diet Dialogue" where

The Easy Weigh Off

many of your questions have been anticipated and then concisely answered. Understanding what nutrients are vital to good health will make you an informed dieter. We'll even have you feeling confident at the checkout counter after you've read hints on how to wisely select your entrees, fruit and vegetables.

So, if you were looking for the "easy weigh off," you've found it! What goes up must come down. As experienced dietitians, we have come in contact with many dieters and as many diet plans. Although our diet is not the only way to lose weight, we feel it is a safe and sensible plan that can be practical and successful for many people. We have selected a wide variety of products for easy availability and enjoyment for the dieter. This plan also accommodates a variety of lifestyles and cooking facilities as well as teaching portion control for formerly "forbidden foods." Being overweight is unhealthy and unnecesary. This diet is simple, well-balanced, great tasting and planned by experts. We think it is *The World's Most Convenient Diet!*

Chapter Two
The Convenience Quotient

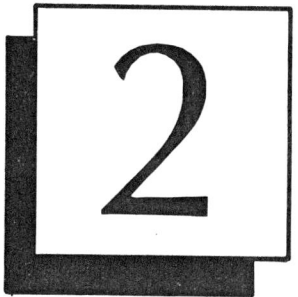

9   Finding Your CQ
9   Convenience Quotient Quiz
10 Scoring
10 Discussion

The Convenience Quotient

Finding Your CQ

The spare tire is there, but the spare time isn't? Your situation is far from unique. Many diets have been sabotaged not by friends or relatives, but by a lack of time. If you consider yourself a busy person, chances are good you have a high CQ. Your CQ is what we call your "Convenience Quotient." It isn't an actual mathematical equation, but if you could hypothetically take the number of pounds you need to lose and divide it by your spare time, you'd end up with a high number. Does that rate you a genius? No, but it does indicate that to get rid of that spare tire without a lot of spare time, you would adhere best to a simple and convenient weight-loss plan.

Convenient Quotient Quiz

We've compiled a list of 10 questions that address concerns which often become obstacles on reduction diets. See if you recognize any of these from your own experience. After reading each question, mark the Yes or No column to the right. After completing the survey, check the scoring and discussion section to decide if *The World's Most Convenient Diet* is for you.

		YES	NO
1.	Do you prefer a variety of foods in a weight-loss diet?		
2.	Would you rather not be bothered with counting calories?		
3.	Do you have a busy lifestyle?		
4.	Do you like meals that are easily prepared?		
5.	Do you enjoy the wide array of convenience foods offered on today's market?		
6.	Do you fear you are limited to buying calorie-reduced products in order to lose or maintain weight?		
7.	Do you find it tedious to weigh and measure portion sizes?		

The World's Most Convenient Diet

	YES	NO
8. Is tasting while cooking a steady source of extra calories in your diet?	____	____
9. Are leftovers difficult for you to ignore?	____	____
10. Do you prefer a well-balanced, three-meals-a-day diet to more restrictive weight-loss plans?	____	____

Scoring

Add the checks you have in the yes column. If you've answered yes to at least five questions, *The World's Most Convenient Diet* is a good choice for you. Removing five potential obstacles in your endeavor to lose weight will be a big help. The closer to 10 questions answered affirmatively, the more your CQ shows this program will be effective for you.* To see why this is true, let's discuss each question.

Discussion

1. Boredom is a common complaint of dieters. *The World's Most Convenient Diet* remedies this by offering a tremendous variety of meals – in fact, more than 300. So that you're not overwhelmed, breakfasts, lunches and dinners are divided into categories that correspond to lifestyles. There are breakfasts that can be popped in a toaster and some that can be prepared in a microwave. Lunches include simple sandwiches to carry to work and hearty soups to enjoy at home. There are meal guidelines for fast food restaurants. You even have the option of preparing meals from scratch on a day you'd like to dirty some pots and pans. So if your answer here is "Yes, variety is important to me," then this diet should work for you.
2. Calculating nutrients – including calories and grams of protein, fat or carbohydrates – can get to be technical. Sometimes the necessary information is not available on package labels. At other times, nutrient data are given in terms of 100-gram servings and most dieters are not aware of the gram size of their serving. An important feature of *The World's Most Convenient Diet* is that all the nutrient calculations – including calories,

---

* Remember to check with your physician before beginning any weight-loss program.

The Convenience Quotient

protein, fat and sodium – have been done beforehand, using the most recent product information available from manufacturers. Following the recommended portion sizes, you should lose weight safely and simply. There's no need to count anything except the pounds you lose.

3. Who doesn't have a busy lifestyle? We all choose different ways to fill our days, with the same end result – not very much extra time! *The World's Most Convenient Diet* will actually create extra time in your day because meal preparation time is minimal. Here's a diet that will help you gain time while you lose weight!

4. If your answer is yes, easily prepared meals are appealing, the convenient weight-loss plan will appeal to you. Recipes, scales and low-calorie cooking techniques are not required. It may come as a surprise to you, but it *is* possible to lose weight eating the same foods as your slim acquaintances do. The key is knowing how to include these meals in a weight-loss plan – and that is done for you in *The World's Most Convenient Diet*.

5. The demand for convenience foods continues to grow, and as a result, the selection is better than ever. Bagels, croissants, lasagna and seafood are all items you can enjoy as you lose weight.

6. Although calorie-reduced products can be part of a reduction diet, they do not need to be. At times the difference between a "light" product and its regular counterpart can be as few as 50 calories. For this reason, many products used on this diet are non-diet items.

7. Getting a little tired of broiling your meat, trimming the fat, dissecting the bone and then weighing what used to be a whole chicken leg? This is another common complaint of dieters. An advantage of most foods allowed on *The World's Most Convenient Diet* is that they are pre-measured. You'll get to enjoy your meal without worrying if the portion size is correct.

8. Too many cooks spoil the broth – to say nothing about too many tastes spoiling the cook! A common source of calories (and pounds) are those extra little meals that result from "just one more taste" during cooking. This temptation is virtually eliminated on *The World's Most Convenient Diet* because most products are packaged and remain sealed during preparation. And besides, you don't have to check your culinary skills – the cooking has already been done.

9. Leftovers will always be a temptation for dieters. We can all relate to Dagwood and his midnight refrigerator raids. To eliminate this obstacle, most entrees selected on *The World's Most Convenient Diet* are specially prepared in single servings – not in amounts suitable for the whole family or neighborhood. You dine knowing the entree you chose is an appropriate meal on your weight-loss plan and there will be no leftovers.

10. If you are discouraged by semi-starvation diets or those that restrict foods to one or two categories, you'll be much happier with the variety this weight-loss program provides. Fish, poultry, meat, milk, cheeses, fruits, vegetables, rolls and pasta can all be part of your daily selection. Three meals a day are required. It is healthier and more effective to spread the nutrients (calories are nutrients) throughout the day.

And Now

Chapter Three
The World's MostConvenient Diet

15	Basic Directions
19	Fresh Fruit Stand
21	Super Salad Bar
22	Free Foods

And Now the World's Most Convenient Diet

Now that you've been introduced to the concept of this convenient diet program, it's time to experience the ease and satisfaction of actual weight loss. First, let's set some rules and definitions to be followed. After that, we'll discuss the Fresh Fruit Stand that lists the choices of fruit to be included with your meals. The vegetables are found in a similar list – the Super Salad Bar, which is followed by the Free Foods. Sample menus are provided to offer examples of how to include these foods in your daily menus.

Basic Directions

1. Choose one breakfast, one lunch and one dinner each day. The choices are found in the Menu Planner beginning in Chapter 5. Once a menu is selected, it must be followed exactly and used for the designated meal only. For example, don't substitute a lunch for a dinner. You may repeat menus, but we suggest varying your choices to keep the diet interesting.

2. Each day, men should include two eight-ounce cups of low-fat milk in addition to any milk that may already be listed in the selected menus. This added milk will guarantee adequate protein levels. The two cups of low-fat milk can be used as snacks or with meals.

   Women have the option of including the two extra cups of low-fat milk. The calorie content of the diet will be increased by approximately 120 calories for each eight-ounce cup.

3. Take one multivitamin-with-minerals tablet each day. We have provided a list of supplements that meet, but do not over-exceed, the Recommended Daily Allowance. The supplement is necessary because even though *The World's Most Convenient Diet* is well balanced, it is sometimes difficult to get enough calcium and iron when calories are restricted. Please note that any additional intake of these supplements is not recommended. That can be a waste of money as well as being potentially harmful.

Although *The World's Most Convenient Diet* requires very little measuring, the following Dieter's Definitions do need attention.

Dieter's Definitions

1 cup	one 8 ounce measuring cup (8 fluid ounces)
¾ cup	¾ of an 8 ounce measuring cup (6 fluid ounces)
½ cup	½ of an 8 ounce measuring cup (4 fluid ounces)
1 tablespoon	1 *level* measuring tablespoon (½ fluid ounce)
1 teaspoon	1 *level* measuring teaspoon
low-fat milk	milk containing 2 percent or less fat. Skim milk may be substituted to further reduce calories.
low-calorie salad dressing	salad dressing containing 35 calories or fewer per tablespoon.
1 slice bread	1 average size slice. (⅔ to 1 ounce) of whole wheat, rye or white bread. French bread should be sliced no thicker than one inch.
1 hard roll	a roll weighing one ounce or less.
1 soda cracker	one 2-by-2 inch square

Additional Tips For Subtracting Pounds

The diet really is that simple! While you are subtracting pounds, here are some more tips to make reducing even easier:

We suggest that you plan your meals in advance. This way shopping can be done less frequently, which will save more time and guarantee the groceries will be on hand when needed. Having menu items readily available also eliminates any excuse for substitutions on the diet. While in the supermarket, note product titles and weights. Use only those products that are specified by the diet.* Manufacturers do vary their products occasionally and a weight discrepancy of one ounce (thirty grams) or less is acceptable. If you do not see a specific product, ask the manager about it. It may be a simple matter, for example, to

---

* In determining product selection, nutrient information was requested from companies during the first quarter of 1984.

And Now the World's Most Convenient Diet

have *Armour®* Beef Burgundy added to the store's inventory if other *Armour®* products are already stocked. Consult "Supermarket Savvy" in Chapter 9 for further shopping tips.

When choosing your meals, you will find that each breakfast, lunch and dinner section in the Menu Planner is divided into sub-categories. If, for example, you like soups for lunch, go to the Hot and Hearty section. If you prefer sandwiches, choose from the Simple Sandwich meals. To make finding your favorite foods even easier, products are listed in alphabetical order – first by brand name and then by product title.

Once you have your food at home, store and prepare it according to menu and package directions. There are two exceptions: Do not add extra fat or salt. This means you should not fry foods unless specified by the directions for a particular menu. A good example would be *Weaver® Rondelets*. Although frying is a preparation option offered in the package's directions, you must choose the alternate method of baking. In addition to saving calories, baking has another advantage over frying. It means easier preparation and clean-up, and this helps keep the diet exactly what it is intended to be – convenient.

Simplify breakfast preparation for the mornings when you would like an egg. Hard-cooked eggs can be made in advance and refrigerated. They can even be stored already peeled if they are kept covered. If you prefer to have your egg cooked just prior to eating, use a non-stick pan. When used in combination with your allowed margarine or a vegetable cooking spray, clean-up is simple. Or, poach your egg. Remember, eggs also can be cooked in a microwave oven.

If you do not have time to completely cook an entree during your lunch break, first cook it at home so that only reheating is necessary at work. For example, bake your lunch the night before at the same time you are heating your supper.

If cooking facilities are not available at your place of employment, be versatile. Soups and casseroles may be heated ahead of time and carried in a thermos. Also, there are menus listing cold sandwiches and meals from fast food restaurants.

Speaking of sandwiches, remember that the raw vegetables from the Super Salad Bar are permitted in unlimited quantities. This can be a real advantage when creating a delicious lunch. For example, the *Louis Rich™* turkey breast sandwich can be made more interesting with lettuce and tomato, not to mention the addition of alfalfa sprouts. Cucumbers, green peppers, celery and cauliflower are just a few vegetables that can make satisfying and nutritious between-meal snacks.

Keep your salads interesting and convenient. Vary the vegetables and low-calorie dressings for new combinations. Make a supply of salad ahead of time so preparation simply involves scooping a cup full of vegetables into a bowl. To store the vegetables, sprinkle with a small amount of water and refrigerate in a plastic container with a tight-fitting lid. Do not add dressing until you are ready to eat your salad.

The use of sugar with cereal is optional. If you prefer to use the allowed sugar in coffee or tea, that is acceptable. Or, you don't need to use it at all, which will bring an even further reduction in calories.

The margarine listed with meals is also optional. Margarine is used instead of butter to help control the amount of cholesterol and saturated fat. If this aspect of the diet is of special interest to you, it is possible to further decrease saturated fats and cholesterol by limiting egg consumption to two or three per week. Choose menus containing fish or skinless poultry. *Stouffer's® Lean Cuisine®* line was designed to control amounts of saturated fat and producers of other products are reportedly addressing this issue. Margarines and other items containing polyunsaturated fats can be identified by their ingredient lists. Select those listing the following liquid vegetable oils as the primary fat source: corn oil, safflower oil, sunflower seed oil, sesame seed oil and cottonseed oil.

To individualize the diet even further, we offer menus without convenience foods. These are for days you feel like cooking or are planning on eating in restaurants.

Here's the basic guide to follow:

Lunch

3	ounces broiled or baked fish or lean meat with fat or skin removed
1	slice whole wheat, rye or white bread
1	teaspoon margarine
1	trip to The Super Salad Bar
1	tablespoon low-calorie dressing
1	choice from The Fresh Fruit stand

Supper

4	ounces broiled or baked fish or lean meat with fat or skin removed
1	slice whole wheat, rye or white bread
1	teaspoon margarine
1	trip to The Super Salad Bar
1	tablespoon low-calorie dressing
1	choice from The Fresh Fruit Stand

And Now the World's Most Convenient Diet

In the Menu Planner, you will find two sections of "expanded" non-convenience meals. Under Lunches, refer to "When You're the Cook," and for Dinners check "Home Cooking."

The Fresh Fruit Stand

Fresh fruit is a good source of both vitamins and fiber. These are important components of *The World's Most Convenient Diet*. Whenever a menu calls for a choice from The Fresh Fruit Stand, select from this list and be sure to follow the specific portion size. Fresh fruits are your best choice, but canned, frozen or dried fruits may be used if they do not contain sugar or syrup. Artificial sweeteners may be added if desired.

Here's a sample breakfast menu that includes a selection from The Fresh Fruit Stand:

¾   cup *General Mills® Cheerios®*
1   teaspoon sugar
½   cup low-fat milk
½   English muffin
1   teaspoon margarine
1   cup fresh strawberries (one choice from The Fresh Fruit Stand)
    artificial sweetener, if desired

Definition of "one serving"

		One serving
Apple		1 small
Apple juice or cider		⅓ cup
Applesauce		½ cup
Apricots:	fresh	2 medium
	dried	4 halves
Banana		½ small
Berries:	blackberries	1 cup
	blueberries	⅔ cup

boysenberries	½ cup
raspberries	1 cup
strawberries	1 cup
Cantaloupe (6-inch diameter)	¼
Cherries	10
Cranberries: (Cooked)	1 cup
Dates	2
Fruit Cocktail	½ cup
Grapefruit	½
Grapefruit juice	½ cup
Grapefruit sections	½ cup
Grape juice	¼ cup
Grapes	12
Honeydew Melon (7-inch diameter)	⅛
Kiwi	1
Mango	½ small
Nectarine	1 medium
Orange	1 medium
Orange juice	½ cup
Orange sections	½ cup
Papaya	⅓ medium
Peach	½ cup or 1 medium
Pear	½ cup or 1 small
Pineapple	½ cup
Pineapple juice	⅓ cup
Plums	2 small or 1 large
Prunes (dried)	2
Prune juice	¼ cup
Raisins	2 tbs.
Rhubarb (cooked)	¾ cup
Tangerine	1 large
Watermelon	1 cup

And Now the World's Most Convenient Diet

The Super Salad Bar

Fresh vegetables are excellent sources of vitamins, minerals and fiber. Whenever a menu calls for a choice from the Super Salad Bar, select from this list. A trip to the Super Salad Bar entitles you to any combination of these raw vegetables in unlimited amounts. If your menu includes dressing, it must be limited to the appropriate serving size.

A serving is one tablespoon of any salad dressing containing 35 or fewer calories per tablespoon. Check the labels. *Henri's*® and several other manufacturers offer selections within this limit.

If you prefer, substitute one teaspoon (not tablespoon) of vegetable oil and unlimited vinegar. Or you may skip dressings and use lemon instead to further reduce the calories.

The Super Salad Bar List

Alfalfa sprouts	Escarole
Asparagus	Kohlrabi
Bamboo shoots	Lettuce (butterhead, cos, iceberg, leaf, romaine)
Bean sprouts	
Beans (snap, green, yellow, wax)	Mushrooms
Broccoli	Onions
Brussels sprouts	Scallions
Cabbage (green, red, Chinese)	Parsley
	Peppers
Carrots	Radishes
Cauliflower	Spinach
Celery	Squash (summer)
Chives	Tomatoes
Cucumber	Watercress
Endive	

Here's an example of how to use a trip to The Super Salad Bar and a choice from The Fresh Fruit Stand to liven up your meal.

Your dinner can go from this –

1   package 11⅔ ounces *Swanson*® *Le Menu*™ Pepper Steak
1   trip to The Super Salad Bar
1   tablespoon low-calorie dressing
1   choice from The Fresh Fruit Stand

To this –

1	package 11⅔ ounces *Swanson® Le Menu*™ Pepper Steak
1	tossed salad containing romaine lettuce, fresh mushrooms, cauliflower and sliced tomato
1	tablespoon *Henri®* Thousand Island Reduced Calorie Dressing
½	cup fresh pineapple chunks

Free Foods

The Free Foods list provides beverages, condiments and spices that contain insignificant amounts of calories. With the exception of ketchup and mustard, free foods may be used in unlimited quantities. Using these items with imagination can make your meals even more varied and enjoyable. Here's an example of what can be done with a menu from the Simple Sandwiches section.

Before adding Free Foods and a visit to the Fresh Fruit Stand:

3	slices *Oscar Mayer®* 95% Fat Free Cooked Ham
2	slices bread
1	trip to the Super Salad Bar
2	choices from the Fresh Fruit Stand

After adding Free Foods and choices from The Fresh Fruit Stand:

3	slices *Oscar Mayer®* 95% Fat Free Cooked Ham topped with lettuce (Free Food) and
1	teaspoon yellow mustard (Free Food)
2	slices fresh rye bread carrot and celery sticks (1 trip to The Super Salad Bar)
1	crisp McIntosh Apple (1 choice from The Fresh Fruit Stand)
1	large plum (1 choice from The Fresh Fruit Stand)

And Now the World's Most Convenient Diet

1 tall glass of iced tea with a lemon wedge (Free Food)

artificial sweetener, if desired (Free Food)

Free Food List

Artificial sweeteners that do not contain sugar, lactose or Sorbitol
Carbonated sugar-free beverages or soda water, mineral water or ice water
Coffee, regular or decaffeinated (without sugar)
Herbs and spices that do not contain sodium or salt
Horseradish
Ketchup, one tablespoon per day
Lemon
Lime
Mustard, brown or yellow, one teaspoon per day
Sugar-free chewing gum
Tea (without sugar)
Vegetables (see Super Salad Bar)
Vinegar

Chapter Four
Seven-Day Sample Plan

27 Shopping Guide For The First Week

29 One-Week Sample Menu

Seven-Day Sample Plan

Shopping Guide For The First Week

This shopping guide is offered for your convenience. It corresponds with the One-Week Sample Menu. There are several items on this list that you can use through the following weeks. Bagels, cereals, muffins, syrup, salad dressings, margarine and eggs are such items. Check and see; you may have some of the listed products at home. Remember to continue making shopping guides for each week you are dieting. Having all the food at your fingertips makes dieting easier.

Dairy

Eggs
Cream cheese
Margarine
Low-fat milk
Yogurt

Breads/Cereals

Bread
French Bread (store in freezer)
Nature Valley® Granola Bars
Kellogg's® *Special K*® Cereal

Meats

Louis Rich™ Oven Roasted Turkey Breast
Fresh Chicken

Frozen Foods

1 pg. (11 oz.)	*Armour Classic Lite*™ Veal Pepper Steak Dinner
1 pkg.	*Aunt Jemima*® Jumbo Buttermilk Waffles
1 pkg. (9 oz.)	*Green Giant*® Lasagna
1 pkg.	*Lender's*® Bagels, any variety
1 pkg.	*Mrs. Paul's*® Light and Natural Sole Fillets
1 pkg.	*Oregon Farms*® Blueberry Crumb Cakes
1 pkg.	*Pepperidge Farm*® Delis, Sliced Beef with Brown Sauce
1 pkg. (9⅝ oz.)	*Stouffer's*® *Lean Cuisine*®

The World's Most Convenient Diet

1 pkg. (312 gms.)	Beef and Pork Cannelloni with Mornay Sauce *Swanson® LeMenu™* Yankee Pot Roast

Canned Goods

Campbell's® Chunky® Clam Chowder, Manhattan Style (19 oz. can)

Condiments, Sauces, Beverages

Aunt Jemima® Lite Syrup Product
Barbeque Sauce (or ingredients for your favorite homemade sauce)
Low-calorie salad dressing
Oil and vinegar for homemade salad dressing
Beverages (diet soda, iced tea, tea, coffee)

Produce

Fresh fruits and vegetables

If you are not planning to use Thursday's fast food option, add a package of sandwich buns and one package of *Weaver®* Chicken Rondelets to your shopping guide.

Seven-Day Sample Plan

One-Week Sample Menu

Monday

Breakfast
1   *Oregon Farms®* Blueberry Crumb Cake
1   cup low-fat milk
1   choice from the Fresh Fruit Stand
1* cup coffee or tea

Lunch
1   Turkey sandwich made with
3   slices *Louis Rich™* Oven Roasted Turkey Breast; top with extras from The Super Salad Bar
2   slices whole wheat, rye or white bread
1   trip to The Super Salad Bar
1   tablespoon low-calorie dressing
2   choices from The Fresh Fruit Stand
1   diet soda or iced tea with lemon

Dinner
1   package (9 oz.) *Green Giant®* Lasagna
1   cup low-fat milk
1   trip to The Super Salad Bar
1   teaspoon oil with unlimited vinegar as dressing
1   choice from The Fresh Fruit Stand
1   cup coffee or tea

Tuesday

Breakfast
¾ cup *Kellogg's® Special K®*
1   teaspoon sugar, optional
½ cup low-fat milk
½ English muffin
1   teaspoon margarine
1   choice from The Fresh Fruit Stand
1   cup coffee or tea

Lunch
1   *Pepperidge Farm Deli®*, Sliced Beef with Brown Sauce
1   trip to The Super Salad Bar
2   choices from The Fresh Fruit Stand
1   diet soda or iced tea with lemon

The World's Most Convenient Diet

Dinner

- 1 package (11 oz.) *Armour® Classic Lite™* Veal Pepper Steak dinner
- 1 slice whole wheat, rye or white bread
- 1 teaspoon margarine
- 1 trip to The Super Salad Bar
- 1 tablespoon low-calorie dressing
- 1 choice from The Fresh Fruit Stand
- 1 cup coffee or tea

Wednesday

Breakfast

- 2 *Aunt Jemima®* Jumbo Buttermilk Waffles
- 3 tablespoons *Aunt Jemima®* Lite Syrup Product
- 1 choice from The Fresh Fruit Stand
- 1 cup coffee or tea

Lunch

- 1 Chef's salad made with
- 3 ounces of lean meat, cut in strips (*Louis Rich™* Oven Roasted Turkey Breast) variety of vegetables from The Super Salad Bar
- 1 tablespoon low-calorie dressing
- 1 slice French bread
- 2 choices from The Fresh Fruit Stand
- 1 diet soda or iced tea with lemon

Dinner

- 1 fillet (6 oz.) *Mrs. Paul's®* Light and Natural Sole Fillets
- 1 slice French bread
- 1 trip to The Super Salad Bar
- 1 tablespoon low-calorie dressing
- 2 choices from The Fresh Fruit Stand
- 1 cup coffee or tea

Seven-Day Sample Plan

Thursday

Breakfast
- 1 *Lender's®* bagel, any variety
- 1 tablespoon cream cheese
- 1 choice from The Fresh Fruit Stand
- ½ cup low-fat milk
- 1 cup coffee or tea

Lunch
- 1 *Wendy's®* Chicken Sandwich
  top with lettuce and tomato
- 1 choice from The Fresh Fruit Stand
- 1 diet soda or iced tea with lemon

or

- 1 *Weaver®* Chicken Rondelet
- 1 sandwich bun
  top with lettuce and tomato
- 1 trip to The Super Salad Bar
- 1 choice from The Fresh Fruit Stand
- 1 diet soda or iced tea with lemon

Dinner
- 1 package (9⅝ oz.) *Stouffer's® Lean Cuisine®* Beef and Pork Cannelloni with Mornay Sauce
- 1 slice whole wheat, rye or white bread
- 1 teaspoon margarine
- 1 trip to The Super Salad Bar
- 1 teaspoon oil with unlimited vinegar as dressing
- 2 choices from The Fresh Fruit Stand
- 1 cup coffee or tea

Friday

Breakfast
- ¾ cup *Kellogg's® Special K®*
- 1 teaspoon sugar, optional
- ½ cup low-fat milk
- ½ English muffin
- 1 teaspoon margarine
- 1 choice from The Fresh Fruit Stand
- 1 cup coffee or tea

The World's Most Convenient Diet

Lunch

- 1 *Pepperidge Farm®* Deli, Sliced Beef with Brown Sauce
- 1 trip to The Super Salad Bar
- 2 choices from The Fresh Fruit Stand
- 1 diet soda or iced tea with lemon

Dinner

- 1 fillet (6 oz.) *Mrs. Paul's®* Light and Natural Sole Fillets
- 1 slice French bread
- 1 trip to The Super Salad Bar
- 1 tablespoon low-calorie dressing
- 2 choices from The Fresh Fruit Stand
- 1 cup coffee or tea

Saturday

Breakfast

- 2 *Aunt Jemima®* Jumbo Buttermilk Waffles
- 3 tablespoons *Aunt Jemima®* Lite Syrup Product
- 1 choice from The Fresh Fruit Stand
- 1 cup coffee or tea

Lunch

- 1 carton (6 to 8 oz.) fruit or flavored yogurt, any brand, including *Bordon's®*, *Dannon®*, *Meadow Gold®*, or *Yoplait®*
- 1 *Nature Valley®* Granola Bar, any variety
- 1 choice from The Fresh Fruit Stand
- 1 diet soda or iced tea with lemon

Dinner

- 1 package (312 grams) *Swanson® Le Menu*™ Yankee Pot Roast
- 1 trip to The Super Salad Bar
- 1 tablespoon low-calorie dressing
- 1 choice from The Fresh Fruit Stand
- 1 cup coffee or tea

Seven-Day Sample Plan

Sunday

Breakfast
- 1 *Oregon Farms®* Blueberry Crumb Cake
- 1 egg, any style prepared without fat
- 1 choice from The Fresh Fruit Stand
- 1 cup coffee or tea

Lunch
- ½ can (19 oz. size) *Campbell's® Chunky®* Clam Chowder Manhattan Style
- 1 cup low-fat milk
- 1 trip to The Super Salad Bar
- 1 teaspoon oil with unlimited vinegar as dressing
- 1 choice from The Fresh Fruit Stand
- 1 diet soda or iced tea with lemon

Dinner
- 4 ounces broiled or grilled barbecued chicken, skin removed
- 2 tablespoons barbecue sauce
- 1 slice French bread
- 1 teaspoon margarine
- 1 trip to The Super Salad Bar
- 1 tablespoon low-calorie dressing
- 1 choice from The Fresh Fruit Stand
- 1 cup coffee or tea

* Note: Although you must follow the milk and food choices in the menus exactly, it isn't necessary to drink specified beverages such as coffee or tea. Those listed are suggestions; you may prefer another. Check the Free Food list for beverages allowed.

Chapter Five
The Menu Planner

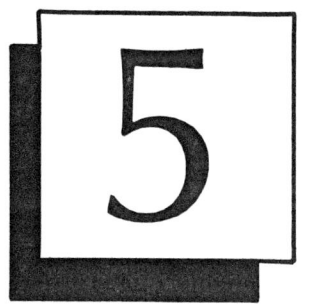

37 Breakfast
59 Lunch
81 Dinner

Breakfast

39	Ready to Eat Cereals
49	Hot Cereals
51	Toaster Breakfasts
53	Bakery Breakfasts
56	Miscellaneous Breakfasts

The Menu Planner

Breakfast

Choice of	**Ready To Eat Cereals**

¾ cup *General Mills® Cheerios®*
1 teaspoon sugar
½ cup low-fat milk
1 slice whole wheat, rye or white toast
  or
½ English muffin
  or
½ bagel, any flavor
1 teaspoon margarine
1 choice from the Fresh Fruit Stand

¾ cup *General Mills® Corn Total®*
½ cup low-fat milk
1 slice whole wheat, rye or white toast
  or
½ English muffin
  or
½ bagel, any flavor
1 teaspoon margarine
1 choice from The Fresh Fruit Stand

½ cup *General Mills® Crispy Wheats 'N Raisins®*
1 teaspoon sugar
½ cup low-fat milk
1 slice whole wheat, rye or white toast
  or
½ English muffin
  or
½ bagel, any flavor
1 teaspoon margarine
1 choice from The Fresh Fruit Stand

¾ cup *General Mills® Kix®*
1 teaspoon sugar
½ cup low-fat milk
1 slice whole wheat, rye or white toast
  or
½ English muffin
  or
½ bagel, any flavor
1 teaspoon margarine
1 choice from The Fresh Fruit Stand

The World's Most Convenient Diet

Breakfast

¾ cup *General Mills® Total®*
1 teaspoon sugar
½ cup low-fat milk
1 slice whole wheat, rye or white toast
    or
½ English muffin
    or
½ bagel, any flavor
1 teaspoon margarine
1 choice from The Fresh Fruit Stand

¾ cup *General Mills® Wheaties®*
1 teaspoon sugar
½ cup low-fat milk
1 slice whole wheat, rye or white toast
    or
½ English muffin
    or
½ bagel, any flavor
1 teaspoon margarine
1 choice from The Fresh Fruit Stand

⅓ cup *Kellogg's® All-Bran®*
1 teaspoon sugar
½ cup low-fat milk
1 slice whole wheat, rye or white toast
    or
½ English muffin
    or
½ bagel, any flavor
1 teaspoon margarine
1 choice from The Fresh Fruit Stand

⅓ cup *Kellogg's® Bran Buds®*
1 teaspoon sugar
½ cup low-fat milk
1 slice whole wheat, rye or white toast
    or
½ English muffin
    or
½ bagel, any flavor
1 teaspoon margarine
1 choice from The Fresh Fruit Stand

The World's Most Convenient Diet

The Menu Planner

Breakfast

⅓ cup *Kellogg's® Cracklin' Oat Bran*™
½ cup low-fat milk
1 slice whole wheat, rye or white toast
   or
½ English muffin
   or
½ bagel, any flavor
1 teaspoon margarine
1 choice from The Fresh Fruit Stand

⅔ cup *Kellogg's® Crispix®*
1 teaspoon sugar
½ cup low-fat milk
1 slice whole wheat, rye or white toast
   or
½ English muffin
   or
½ bagel, any flavor
1 teaspoon margarine
1 choice from The Fresh Fruit Stand

---

3 biscuits *Kellogg's® Frosted Mini-Wheats®*
   (sugar-frosted or brown sugar-cinnamon flavor)
½ cup low-fat milk
1 slice whole wheat, rye or white toast
   or
½ English muffin
   or
½ bagel, any flavor
1 teaspoon margarine
1 choice from The Fresh Fruit Stand

⅓ cup *Kellogg's® Frosted Krispies*™
½ cup low-fat milk
1 slice whole wheat, rye or white toast
   or
½ English muffin
   or
½ bagel, any flavor
1 teaspoon margarine
1 choice from The Fresh Fruit Stand

The World's Most Convenient Diet

Breakfast

½ cup *Kellogg's® Fruitful Bran*™
½ cup low-fat milk
1 slice whole wheat, rye or white toast
    or
½ English muffin
    or
½ bagel, any flavor
1 teaspoon margarine
1 choice from The Fresh Fruit Stand

½ cup *Kellogg's® Honey & Nut Cornflakes*™
½ cup low-fat milk
1 slice whole wheat, rye or white toast
    or
½ English muffin
    or
½ bagel, any flavor
1 teaspoon margarine
1 choice from The Fresh Fruit Stand

⅓ cup *Kellogg's® Most®*
1 teaspoon sugar
½ cup low-fat milk
1 slice whole wheat, rye or white toast
    or
½ English muffin
    or
½ bagel, any flavor
1 teaspoon margarine
1 choice from The Fresh Fruit Stand

⅓ cup *Kellogg's® Nutri·Grain®*, Corn, Wheat or Wheat & Raisins
1 teaspoon sugar
½ cup low-fat milk
1 slice whole wheat, rye or white toast
    or
½ English muffin
    or
½ bagel, any flavor
1 teaspoon margarine
1 choice from The Fresh Fruit Stand

The Menu Planner

Breakfast

⅓ cup *Kellogg's® Product 19®*
1 teaspoon sugar
½ cup low-fat milk
1 slice whole wheat, rye or white toast
   or
½ English muffin
   or
½ bagel, any flavor
1 teaspoon margarine
1 choice from The Fresh Fruit Stand

⅓ cup *Kellogg's® Raisins, Rice and Rye™*
1 teaspoon sugar
½ cup low-fat milk
1 slice whole wheat, rye or white toast
   or
½ English muffin
   or
½ bagel, any flavor
1 teaspoon margarine
1 choice from The Fresh Fruit Stand

¾ cup *Kellogg's® Rice Krispies®*
1 teaspoon sugar
½ cup low-fat milk
1 slice whole wheat, rye or white toast
   or
½ English muffin
   or
½ bagel, any flavor
1 teaspoon margarine
1 choice from The Fresh Fruit Stand

¾ cup *Kellogg's® Special K®*
1 teaspoon sugar
½ cup low-fat milk
1 slice whole wheat, rye or white toast
   or
½ English muffin
   or
½ bagel, any flavor
1 teaspoon margarine
1 choice from The Fresh Fruit Stand

The World's Most Convenient Diet

Breakfast

½ cup *Nabisco*® 100% Bran Cereal
1 teaspoon sugar
½ cup low-fat milk
1 slice whole wheat, rye or white toast
    or
½ English muffin
    or
½ bagel, any flavor
1 teaspoon margarine
1 choice from The Fresh Fruit Stand

---

1 biscuit, *Nabisco*® Shredded Wheat
1 teaspoon sugar
½ cup low-fat milk
1 slice whole wheat, rye or white toast
    or
½ English muffin
    or
½ bagel, any flavor
1 teaspoon margarine
1 choice from The Fresh Fruit Stand

⅔ cup *Nabisco*® *Spoon Size*® Shredded Wheat
1 teaspoon sugar
½ cup low-fat milk
1 slice whole wheat, rye or white toast
    or
½ English muffin
    or
½ bagel, any flavor
1 teaspoon margarine
1 choice from The Fresh Fruit Stand

¾ cup *Nabisco*® *Team*® Flakes Cereal
1 teaspoon sugar
½ cup low-fat milk
1 slice whole wheat, rye or white toast
    or
½ English muffin
    or
½ bagel, any flavor
1 teaspoon margarine
1 choice from The Fresh Fruit Stand

The Menu Planner

Breakfast

½ cup *Post® Grape-Nuts®* Flakes
1 teaspoon sugar
½ cup low-fat milk
1 slice whole wheat, rye or white toast
   or
½ English muffin
   or
½ bagel, any flavor
1 teaspoon margarine
1 choice from The Fresh Fruit Stand

½ cup *Post®* Fortified Oat Flakes
1 teaspoon sugar
½ cup low-fat milk
1 slice whole wheat, rye or white toast
   or
½ English muffin
   or
½ bagel, any flavor
1 teaspoon margarine
1 choice from The Fresh Fruit Stand

½ cup, *Quaker®* Corn Bran
½ cup low-fat milk
1 slice whole wheat, rye or white toast
   or
½ English muffin
   or
½ bagel, any flavor
1 teaspoon margarine
1 choice from The Fresh Fruit Stand

½ cup *Quaker® Cinnamon Life®*
½ cup low-fat milk
1 slice whole wheat, rye or white toast
   or
½ English muffin
   or
½ bagel, any flavor
1 teaspoon margarine
1 choice from The Fresh Fruit Stand

The World's Most Convenient Diet

Breakfast

½ cup *Quaker® Life®* Cereal
½ cup low-fat milk
1 slice whole wheat, rye or white toast
  or
½ English muffin
  or
½ bagel, any flavor
1 teaspoon margarine
1 choice from The Fresh Fruit Stand

---

1 cup *Quaker®* Puffed Rice
1 teaspoon sugar
½ cup low-fat milk
1 slice whole wheat, rye or white toast
  or
½ English muffin
  or
½ bagel, any flavor
1 teaspoon margarine
1 choice from The Fresh Fruit Stand

---

1 cup *Quaker®* Puffed Wheat
1 teaspoon sugar
½ cup low-fat milk
1 slice whole wheat, rye or white toast
  or
½ English muffin
  or
½ bagel, any flavor
1 teaspoon margarine
1 choice from The Fresh Fruit Stand

---

1 biscuit *Quaker®* Shredded Wheat
1 teaspoon sugar
½ cup low-fat milk
1 slice whole wheat, rye or white toast
  or
½ English muffin
  or
½ bagel, any flavor
1 teaspoon margarine
1 choice from The Fresh Fruit Stand

The Menu Planner

Breakfast

½ cup *Ralston® Bran Chex®*
1 teaspoon sugar
½ cup low-fat milk
1 slice whole wheat, rye or white toast
   or
½ English muffin
   or
½ bagel, any flavor
1 teaspoon margarine
1 choice from The Fresh Fruit Stand

¾ cup *Ralston® Corn Chex®*
1 teaspoon sugar
½ cup low-fat milk
1 slice whole wheat, rye or white toast
   or
½ English muffin
   or
½ bagel, any flavor
1 teaspoon margarine
1 choice from The Fresh Fruit Stand

¾ cup *Ralston® Crispy Rice®*
1 teaspoon sugar
½ cup low-fat milk
1 slice whole wheat, rye or white toast
   or
½ English muffin
   or
½ bagel, any flavor
1 teaspoon margarine
1 choice from The Fresh Fruit Stand

¾ cup *Ralston® Rice Chex®*
1 teaspoon sugar
½ cup low-fat milk
1 slice whole wheat, rye or white toast
   or
½ English muffin
   or
½ bagel, any flavor
1 teaspoon margarine
1 choice from The Fresh Fruit Stand

The World's Most Convenient Diet

Breakfast

¾ cup *Ralston® Tasteeos®*
1 teaspoon sugar
½ cup low-fat milk
1 slice whole wheat, rye or white toast
    or
½ English muffin
    or
½ bagel, any flavor
1 teaspoon margarine
1 choice from The Fresh Fruit Stand

½ cup *Ralston®* Wheat Chex®
1 teaspoon sugar
½ cup low-fat milk
1 slice whole wheat, rye or white toast
    or
½ English muffin
    or
½ bagel, any flavor
1 teaspoon margarine
1 choice from The Fresh Fruit Stand

½ cup *Ralston® Wheat and Raisin Chex®*
1 teaspoon sugar
½ cup low-fat milk
1 slice whole wheat, rye or white toast
    or
½ English muffin
    or
½ bagel, any flavor
1 teaspoon margarine
1 choice from The Fresh Fruit Stand

½ cup 40% bran cereal, any brand
1 teaspoon sugar
½ cup low-fat milk
1 slice whole wheat, rye or white toast
    or
½ English muffin
    or
½ bagel, any flavor
1 teaspoon margarine
1 choice from The Fresh Fruit Stand

The Menu Planner

Breakfast

⠀⠀⠀¾ cup cornflakes, any brand
⠀⠀⠀1 teaspoon sugar
⠀⠀⠀½ cup low-fat milk
⠀⠀⠀1 slice whole wheat, rye or white toast
⠀⠀⠀⠀⠀⠀or
⠀⠀⠀½ English muffin
⠀⠀⠀⠀⠀⠀or
⠀⠀⠀½ bagel, any flavor
⠀⠀⠀1 teaspoon margarine
⠀⠀⠀1 choice from The Fresh Fruit Stand

⠀⠀⠀½ cup raisin bran, any brand
⠀⠀⠀1 teaspoon sugar
⠀⠀⠀½ cup low-fat milk
⠀⠀⠀1 slice whole wheat, rye or white toast
⠀⠀⠀⠀⠀⠀or
⠀⠀⠀½ English muffin
⠀⠀⠀⠀⠀⠀or
⠀⠀⠀½ bagel, any flavor
⠀⠀⠀1 teaspoon margarine
⠀⠀⠀1 choice from The Fresh Fruit Stand

Choice of ⠀⠀⠀**Hot Cereals**

⠀⠀⠀1 packet *Nabisco® Mix 'N Eat Cream of Wheat®* Cereal, Apple 'n Cinnamon flavor
⠀⠀⠀½ cup low-fat milk
⠀⠀⠀1 choice from The Fresh Fruit Stand

⠀⠀⠀1 packet *Nabisco® Mix 'N Eat Cream of Wheat®* Cereal, Brown Sugar Cinnamon flavor
⠀⠀⠀½ cup low-fat milk
⠀⠀⠀1 choice from The Fresh Fruit Stand

⠀⠀⠀1 packet *Nabisco® Mix 'N Eat Cream of Wheat®* Cereal, Honey Graham flavor
⠀⠀⠀½ cup low-fat milk
⠀⠀⠀1 choice from The Fresh Fruit Stand

The World's Most Convenient Diet

Breakfast

1	packet *Nabisco® Mix'N Eat Cream of Wheat®* Cereal, Hot Chocolate flavor
½	cup low-fat milk
1	choice from The Fresh Fruit Stand

1	packet *Nabisco® Mix'N Eat Cream of Wheat®* Cereal, Maple Brown Sugar flavor
½	cup low-fat milk
1	choice from The Fresh Fruit Stand

1	packet *Nabisco® Mix'N Eat Cream of Wheat®* Cereal, original flavor
1	teaspoon white or brown sugar
1	teaspoon margarine
½	cup low-fat milk
1	choice from The Fresh Fruit Stand

1	packet *Nabisco® Mix'N Eat Cream of Wheat®* Cereal, Raisins 'n Spice flavor
½	cup low-fat milk
1	choice from The Fresh Fruit Stand

1	packet Instant *Quaker®* Oatmeal with Apples & Cinnamon flavor
½	cup low-fat milk
1	choice from The Fresh Fruit Stand

1	packet Instant *Quaker®* Oatmeal with Bran & Raisins flavor
½	cup low-fat milk
1	choice from The Fresh Fruit Stand

1	packet Instant *Quaker®* Oatmeal, Cinnamon & Spice flavor
½	cup low-fat milk
1	choice from The Fresh Fruit Stand

The Menu Planner

Breakfast

1	packet Instant *Quaker*® Oatmeal, Honey & Graham flavor
½	cup low-fat milk
1	choice from The Fresh Fruit Stand

1	packet Instant *Quaker*® Oatmeal, Maple & Brown Sugar flavor
½	cup low-fat milk
1	choice from The Fresh Fruit Stand

1	packet Instant *Quaker*® Oatmeal, Raisins & Spice flavor
½	cup low-fat milk
1	choice from The Fresh Fruit Stand

1	packet Instant *Quaker*® Oatmeal, regular flavor
1	teaspoon white or brown sugar
1	teaspoon margarine
½	cup low-fat milk
1	choice from The Fresh Fruit Stand

Choice of   **Toaster Breakfasts**

2	slices *Aunt Jemima*® Cinnamon Swirl French Toast
3	tablespoons *Aunt Jemima*® Lite Syrup Product
1	choice from The Fresh Fruit Stand

2	slices *Aunt Jemima*® French Toast
3	tablespoons *Aunt Jemima*® Lite Syrup Product
1	choice from The Fresh Fruit Stand

2	*Aunt Jemima*® Jumbo Apple & Cinnamon Waffles
3	tablespoons *Aunt Jemima*® Lite Syrup Product
1	choice from The Fresh Fruit Stand

2	*Aunt Jemima*® Jumbo Blueberry Waffles
3	tablespoons *Aunt Jemima*® Lite Syrup Product
1	choice from The Fresh Fruit Stand

The World's Most Convenient Diet

Breakfast

2	*Aunt Jemima*® Jumbo Buttermilk Waffles
3	tablespoons *Aunt Jemima*® Lite Syrup Product
1	choice from The Fresh Fruit Stand

2	*Aunt Jemima*® Jumbo Original Waffles
3	tablespoons *Aunt Jemima*® Lite Syrup Product
1	choice from The Fresh Fruit Stand

1	*Eggo*® Brand Homestyle Waffles Apple Cinnamon
2	tablespoons *Aunt Jemima*® Lite Syrup Product
1	choice from The Fresh Fruit Stand
½	cup low-fat milk

1	*Eggo*® Brand Homestyle Waffles Blueberry
2	tablespoons *Aunt Jemima*® Lite Syrup Product
1	choice from The Fresh Fruit Stand
½	cup low-fat milk

1	*Eggo*® Brand Homestyle Waffles Buttermilk
2	tablespoons *Aunt Jemima*® Lite Syrup Product
1	choice from The Fresh Fruit Stand

1	*Eggo*® Brand Homestyle Waffle
2	tablespoons *Aunt Jemima*® Lite Syrup Product
1	choice from The Fresh Fruit Stand
½	cup low-fat milk

1	*Eggo*® Brand Homestyle Waffles Strawberry
2	tablespoons *Aunt Jemima*® Lite Syrup Product
1	choice from The Fresh Fruit Stand
½	cup low-fat milk

1	*Lender's*® Bagel, any variety
1	tablespoon cream cheese
1	choice from The Fresh Fruit Stand
½	cup low-fat milk

The Menu Planner

Breakfast

1	*Lender's®* Bagel, any variety
1	tablespoon peanut butter
1	choice from The Fresh Fruit Stand

1	*Wonder® Raisin Round®*
1	tablespoon peanut butter
1	choice from The Fresh Fruit Stand

1	English Muffin, any brand including *Bays®*, *Thomas'®* and *Wonder®*
1	tablespoon peanut butter
1	choice from The Fresh Fruit Stand

Choice of

Bakery Breakfasts

1	*Hostess®* Cinnamon Donut
1	egg, any style prepared without fat
	or
1	cup low-fat milk
1	choice from The Fresh Fruit Stand

1	*Hostess®* Plain Donut
1	egg, any style prepared without fat
	or
1	cup low-fat milk
1	choice from The Fresh Fruit Stand

1	*Hostess®* Powdered Sugar Donut
1	egg, any style prepared without fat
	or
1	cup low-fat milk
1	choice from The Fresh Fruit Stand

1	*Hostess®* Blueberry Muffin
1	egg, any style prepared without fat
	or
1	cup low-fat milk
1	choice from The Fresh Fruit Stand

1	*King's Hawaiian®* Original Roll
	or

continued

The World's Most Convenient Diet

Breakfast

1	slice (1 oz.) *King's Hawaiian*® Bread
1	teaspoon margarine
1	egg, any style prepared without fat
	or
1	cup low-fat milk
1	choice from The Fresh Fruit Stand

1	*Morton*® *Donut Shop*® Chocolate Iced Donut
1	cup low-fat milk
1	choice from The Fresh Fruit Stand

1	*Morton*® *Donut Shop*® Glazed Donut
1	cup low-fat milk
1	choice from The Fresh Fruit Stand

1	*Morton*® *Donut Shop*® Mini Donut
1	cup low-fat milk
1	choice from The Fresh Fruit Stand

1	*Morton*® Mini Honey Bun
1	egg, any style prepared without fat
	or
1	cup low-fat milk
1	choice from The Fresh Fruit Stand

1	*Morton*® Blueberry Muffin
1	egg, any style prepared without fat
	or
1	cup low-fat milk
1	choice from The Fresh Fruit Stand

1	*Morton*® Corn Muffin
1	egg, any style prepared without fat
	or
1	cup low-fat milk
1	choice from The Fresh Fruit Stand

1	*Oregon Farms*® Blueberry Crumb Cake
½	cup low-fat milk
1	choice from The Fresh Fruit Stand

The Menu Planner

Breakfast

    1   *Oregon Farms*® Cheese Crumb Cake
    ½   cup low-fat milk
    1   choice from The Fresh Fruit Stand

---

    1   *Oregon Farms*® Cherry Crumb Cake
    ½   cup low-fat milk
    1   choice from The Fresh Fruit Stand

---

    1   *Oregon Farms*® French Crumb Cake
    ½   cup low-fat milk
    1   choice from The Fresh Fruit Stand

---

    1   *Pepperidge Farm*® Old Fashioned Blueberry Muffin
    ½   cup low-fat milk
    1   choice from The Fresh Fruit Stand

---

    1   *Pepperidge Farm*® Old Fashioned Bran with Raisin Muffin
    ½   cup low-fat milk
    1   choice from The Fresh Fruit Stand

---

    1   *Pepperidge Farm*® Old Fashioned Carrot Walnut Muffin
    ½   cup low-fat milk
    1   choice from The Fresh Fruit Stand

---

    1   *Pepperidge Farm*® Old Fashioned Cinnamon Swirl Muffin
    ½   cup low-fat milk
    1   choice from The Fresh Fruit Stand

---

    1   *Pepperidge Farm*® Old Fashioned Corn Muffin
    ½   cup low-fat milk
    1   choice from The Fresh Fruit Stand

---

    1   *Pepperidge Farm*® Old Fashioned Orange-Cranberry Muffin
    ½   cup low-fat milk
    1   choice from The Fresh Fruit Stand

---

    1   *Sara Lee Croissant*®, All Butter flavor   *continued*

The World's Most Convenient Diet

Breakfast

½	cup low-fat milk
1	choice from The Fresh Fruit Stand

1	*Sara Lee Croissant*®, Cheese flavor
½	cup low-fat milk
1	choice from The Fresh Fruit Stand

1	*Sara Lee Croissant*®, Wheat and Honey flavor
½	cup low-fat milk
1	choice from The Fresh Fruit Stand

Choice of

Miscellaneous Breakfasts

½	cup cottage cheese, any brand
1	slice whole wheat, rye or white toast
	or
½	English muffin
	or
½	bagel, any flavor
1	teaspoon margarine
1	choice from The Fresh Fruit Stand

1	egg, any style prepared with
1	teaspoon margarine
1	slice whole wheat, rye or white toast
	or
½	English muffin
	or
½	bagel, any flavor
2	teaspoons any flavor jelly
1	choice from The Fresh Fruit Stand

1	*Nature Valley*® Granola Bar, Almond, Coconut, Cinnamon, Oats 'n Honey or Peanut flavor
1	cup low-fat milk
1	choice from The Fresh Fruit Stand

1	*Nature Valley*® Chewy Granola Bar, Apple or Raisin flavor
1	cup low-fat milk
1	choice from The Fresh Fruit Stand

The Menu Planner

Breakfast

1	*Nature Valley® Granola Clusters®* Roll
1	cup low-fat milk
1	choice from The Fresh Fruit Stand

1	*Nature Valley® Granola & Fruit Bar®*, Apple, Date or Raspberry flavor
1	cup low-fat milk
1	choice from The Fresh Fruit Stand

1	*Quaker™* Chewy Granola Bar, any variety
1	cup low-fat milk
1	choice from The Fresh Fruit Stand

1	carton (6 to 8 oz.) fruit or flavored yogurt, any brand, including *Borden's®*, *Dannon®*, *Meadow Gold®* or *Yoplait®*
1	choice from The Fresh Fruit Stand

1	carton (6 to 8 oz.) plain yogurt, any brand, including *Borden's®*, *Dannon®*, *Meadow Gold®* or *Yoplait®*
1	slice whole wheat, rye or white toast
	or
½	English muffin
	or
½	bagel, any flavor
1	teaspoon margarine
1	choice from The Fresh Fruit Stand

1	carton (6 oz.) *Yoplait® Breakfast Yogurt™*, any flavor
1	choice from The Fresh Fruit Stand

The World's Most Convenient Diet

Lunch

61	Fast Food Fare
62	Simple Sandwiches
66	Hot and Hearty
79	When You're the Cook

The Menu Planner

Lunch

Choice of Fast Food Fare

Remember to be accurate when ordering these items. A *McDonald's®* cheeseburger is not a *Big Mac®* or a double cheeseburger. Be specific and don't add extra sauces. Bring your fresh fruit from home.

1	*Arby's®* French Dip
1	choice from The Fresh Fruit Stand

1	*Arby's®* Regular Roast Beef Sandwich, no sauce
1	choice from The Fresh Fruit Stand

1	*Burger King®* Hamburger with tomato, lettuce or onions
1	trip to the Super Salad Bar
1	tablespoon low-calorie dressing
1	choice from The Fresh Fruit Stand

1	*Dairy Queen Brazier®* Single Hamburger
1	choice from The Fresh Fruit Stand

1	*Kentucky Fried Chicken®* Drumstick
1	serving mashed potatoes with gravy
2	choices from The Fresh Fruit Stand

1	*McDonald's®* Cheeseburger
2	choices from The Fresh Fruit Stand

1	*Taco Bell® Bellbeefer®*
2	choices from The Fresh Fruit Stand

1	*Taco Bell® Bellbeefer®* with Cheese
2	choices from The Fresh Fruit Stand

1	*Wendy's®* Chicken a la King Hot Stuffed Baked Potato
1	choice from The Fresh Fruit Stand

1	*Wendy's®* Chicken Sandwich top with lettuce and tomato

continued

The World's Most Convenient Diet

Lunch

1	choice from The Fresh Fruit Stand

1	8-ounce serving *Wendy's®* Chili
1	trip to the Super Salad Bar
1	tablespoon low-calorie dressing
1	choice from The Fresh Fruit Stand

Choice of **Simple Sandwiches**

½	can (7½ oz. size) *Carnation® The Spreadables®*, Tuna Salad top with extras from The Super Salad Bar
2	slices whole wheat, rye or white bread
1	choice from The Fresh Fruit Stand

½	can (7½ oz. size) *Carnation® The Spreadables®*, Turkey Salad top with extras from The Super Salad Bar
2	slices whole wheat, rye or white bread
1	choice from The Fresh Fruit Stand

2	slices *Eckrich® Calorie Watcher™* Breast of Chicken top with extras from The Super Salad Bar
2	slices whole wheat, rye or white bread
1	trip to The Super Salad Bar
1	teaspoon oil with unlimited vinegar as dressing
2	choices from The Fresh Fruit Stand

2	slices *Eckrich® Calorie Watcher™* Slender Sliced Corned Beef top with extras from The Super Salad Bar
2	slices whole wheat, rye or white bread
1	trip to The Super Salad Bar
1	tablespoon low-calorie dressing
2	choices from The Fresh Fruit Stand

2	slices *Eckrich® Calorie Watcher™* Chopped Ham top with extras from The Super Salad Bar
2	slices whole wheat, rye or white bread
1	trip to The Super Salad Bar

continued

The Menu Planner

Lunch

1	tablespoon low-calorie dressing
2	choices from The Fresh Fruit Stand

2	slices *Eckrich® Calorie Watcher™* Sliced Cooked Ham
	top with extras from The Super Salad Bar
2	slices whole wheat, rye or white bread
1	trip to The Super Salad Bar
1	teaspoon oil with unlimited vinegar as dressing
2	choices from The Fresh Fruit Stand

2	slices *Eckrich® Calorie Watcher™* Sweet Smoked Ham
	top with extras from The Super Salad Bar
2	slices whole wheat, rye or white bread
1	trip to The Super Salad Bar
1	tablespoon low-calorie dressing
2	choices from The Fresh Fruit Stand

2	slices *Eckrich® Calorie Watcher™* Slender Sliced Pastrami
	top with extras from The Super Salad Bar
2	slices whole wheat, rye or white bread
1	trip to The Super Salad Bar
1	tablespoon low-calorie dressing
2	choices from The Fresh Fruit Stand

2	slices *Eckrich® Calorie Watcher™* Slender Sliced Smoked Turkey
	top with extras from The Super Salad Bar
2	slices whole wheat, rye or white bread
1	trip to The Super Salad Bar
1	tablespoon low-calorie dressing
2	choices from The Fresh Fruit Stand

3	slices *Louis Rich™* Turkey Cotto Salami
	top with extras from The Super Salad Bar
2	slices whole wheat, rye or white bread
1	trip to The Super Salad Bar
2	choices from The Fresh Fruit Stand

The World's Most Convenient Diet

Lunch

2	slices *Louis Rich*™ Turkey Ham
	top with extras from The Super Salad Bar
2	slices whole wheat, rye or white bread
1	trip to The Super Salad Bar
1	tablespoon low-calorie dressing
2	choices from The Fresh Fruit Stand

2	slices *Louis Rich*™ Turkey Pastrami
	top with extras from The Super Salad Bar
2	slices whole wheat, rye or white bread
1	trip to The Super Salad Bar
1	tablespoon low-calorie dressing
2	choices from The Fresh Fruit Stand

3	slices *Louis Rich*™ Oven Roasted Turkey Breast
	top with extras from The Super Salad Bar
2	slices whole wheat, rye or white bread
1	trip to The Super Salad Bar
1	tablespoon low-calorie dressing
2	choices from The Fresh Fruit Stand

3	slices *Louis Rich*™ Smoked Turkey Breast
	top with extras from The Super Salad Bar
2	slices whole wheat, rye or white bread
1	trip to The Super Salad Bar
1	tablespoon low-calorie dressing
2	choices from The Fresh Fruit Stand

2	slices *Oscar Mayer*® 90% Fat Free Bar-B-Q Loaf
	top with extras from The Super Salad Bar
2	slices whole wheat, rye or white bread
1	trip to The Super Salad Bar
1	tablespoon low-calorie dressing
2	choices from The Fresh Fruit Stand

2	slices *Oscar Mayer*® 93% Fat Free Canadian Style Bacon
	top with extras from The Super Salad Bar
2	slices whole wheat, rye or white bread
1	trip to The Super Salad Bar
1	tablespoon low-calorie dressing
2	choices from The Fresh Fruit Stand

The Menu Planner

Lunch

3	slices *Oscar Mayer*® 95% Fat Free Cooked Ham top with extras from The Super Salad Bar
2	slices whole wheat, rye or white bread
1	trip to The Super Salad Bar
1	teaspoon oil with unlimited vinegar as dressing
2	choices from The Fresh Fruit Stand

2	slices *Oscar Mayer*® 93% Fat Free Peppered Loaf top with extras from The Super Salad Bar
2	slices whole wheat, rye or white bread
1	trip to The Super Salad Bar
1	tablespoon low-calorie dressing
2	choices from The Fresh Fruit Stand

½	can (6 or 7 oz. size) water-packed tuna (any brand including *Bumble Bee*®, *Chicken of the Sea*® or *Star-Kist*®) mixed with
1	tablespoon mayonnaise or salad dressing, chopped onion, celery and green pepper served on
2	slices whole wheat, rye or white bread
1	choice from The Fresh Fruit Stand

½	can (4¾ oz. size) *Underwood*® Chunky Chicken Spread top with extras from The Super Salad Bar
2	slices whole wheat, rye or white bread
1	trip to The Super Salad Bar
2	choices from The Fresh Fruit Stand

½	can (4¾ oz. size) *Underwood*® Roast Beef Spread top with extras from The Super Salad Bar
2	slices whole wheat, rye or white bread
1	trip to The Super Salad Bar
2	choices from The Fresh Fruit Stand

1	6 or 8 oz. carton fruit or flavored yogurt, any brand including *Bordon's*®, *Dannon*®, *Meadow Gold*® or *Yoplait*®
1	*Nature Valley Granola Bar*®, any variety or *Quaker*® Chewy Granola Bar, any variety
1	choice from The Fresh Fruit Stand

The World's Most Convenient Diet

Lunch

Choice of		Hot and Hearty
	1	package (10 oz.) *Armour Classic Lite*™ Beef Pepper Steak
	1	trip to The Super Salad Bar
	1	tablespoon low-calorie dressing
	1	choice from The Fresh Fruit Stand
	1	package (11¼ oz.) *Armour Classic Lite*™ Chicken Burgundy
	1	trip to The Super Salad Bar
	1	tablespoon low-calorie dressing
	1	choice from The Fresh Fruit Stand
	1	package (10 oz.) *Armour Classic Lite*™ Chicken Oriental
	1	trip to The Super Salad Bar
	1	tablespoon low-calorie dressing
	1	choice from The Fresh Fruit Stand
	1	package (13¼ oz.) *Armour Classic Lite*™ Filet of Cod Divan
	1	trip to The Super Salad Bar
	1	tablespoon low-calorie dressing
	1	choice from The Fresh Fruit Stand
	1	package (10 oz.) *Armour Classic Lite*™ Turf and Surf
	1	trip to The Super Salad Bar
	1	tablespoon low-calorie dressing
	1	choice from The Fresh Fruit Stand
	1	package (11 oz.) *Armour Classic Lite*™ Turkey Parmesan
	1	trip to The Super Salad Bar
	1	tablespoon low-calorie dressing
	1	choice from The Fresh Fruit Stand
	1	package (11 oz.) *Armour Classic Lite*™ Veal Pepper Steak
	1	trip to The Super Salad Bar

continued

The Menu Planner

Lunch

1	tablespoon low-calorie dressing
1	choice from The Fresh Fruit Stand

1	package (10½ oz.) *Armour Dinner Classic*® Beef Burgundy
1	choice from The Fresh Fruit Stand

1	package (11¼ oz.) *Armour Dinner Classic*® Beef Stroganoff
1	choice from The Fresh Fruit Stand

1	package (11¾ oz.) *Armour Dinner Classic*® Chicken Fricassee
1	choice from The Fresh Fruit Stand

1	package (12 oz.) *Armour Dinner Classic*® Cod Almondine
1	choice from The Fresh Fruit Stand

1	*Armour*® Turkey Frank
1	hot dog bun
1	cup low-fat milk
1	choice from The Fresh Fruit Stand

1	cup *B & M*® Red Kidney, Small Pea or Yellow Eye Baked Beans
1	trip to The Super Salad Bar
1	choice from The Fresh Fruit Stand

1	package (5 oz.) *Banquet*® Cookin' Bag Chicken Ala King
1	sandwich bun, open-faced
1	trip to The Super Salad Bar
1	tablespoon low-calorie dressing
1	choice from The Fresh Fruit Stand

1	package (8 oz.) *Banquet*® Spaghetti with Meat Sauce
1	trip to The Super Salad Bar
1	teaspoon oil with unlimited vinegar as dressing
1	choice from The Fresh Fruit Stand

The World's Most Convenient Diet

Lunch

1	can (7⅞ oz.) *Campbell's® Beans and Franks*
1	choice from The Fresh Fruit Stand

1	can (11 oz.) *Campbell's® Chunky®* Old Fashioned Bean with Ham Soup
1	trip to The Super Salad Bar
1	teaspoon oil with unlimited vinegar as dressing
2	choices from The Fresh Fruit Stand

½	can (19¼ oz. size) *Campbell's® Chunky®* Old Fashioned Bean with Ham Soup
1	cup low-fat milk
1	choice from The Fresh Fruit Stand

1	can (10¾ oz.) *Campbell's® Chunky®* Beef Soup
1	trip to The Super Salad Bar
1	teaspoon oil with unlimited vinegar as dressing
2	choices from The Fresh Fruit Stand

½	can (19 oz. size) *Campbell's® Chunky®* Beef Soup
1	trip to The Super Salad Bar
1	teaspoon oil with unlimited vinegar as dressing
2	choices from The Fresh Fruit Stand

1	can (10¾ oz. size) *Campbell's® Chunky®* Chicken Soup
1	trip to The Super Salad Bar
1	teaspoon oil with unlimited vinegar as dressing
2	choices from The Fresh Fruit Stand

1	can (11 oz.) *Campbell's® Chunky®* Chili Beef Soup
1	trip to The Super Salad Bar
1	teaspoon oil with unlimited vinegar as dressing
1	choice from The Fresh Fruit Stand

½	can (19½ oz.) *Campbell's® Chunky®* Chili Beef Soup
1	trip to The Super Salad Bar
1	teaspoon oil with unlimited vinegar as dressing
2	choices from The Fresh Fruit Stand

The Menu Planner

Lunch

½ can (19 oz. size) *Campbell's® Chunky®* Clam Chowder (Manhattan Style)
1 cup low-fat milk
1 trip to The Super Salad Bar
1 teaspoon oil with unlimited vinegar as dressing
1 choice from The Fresh Fruit Stand

½ can (19 oz. size) *Campbell's® Chunky®* Mediterranean Vegetable Soup
1 cup low-fat milk
1 trip to The Super Salad Bar
1 choice from The Fresh Fruit Stand

½ can (19½ oz. size) *Campbell's® Chunky®* Mexicali Bean Soup
1 cup low-fat milk
1 trip to The Super Salad Bar
1 choice from The Fresh Fruit Stand

---

1 can (10¾ oz. size) *Campbell's® Chunky®* Split Pea with Ham Soup
1 trip to The Super Salad Bar
1 teaspoon oil with unlimited vinegar as dressing
2 choices from The Fresh Fruit Stand

½ can (19 oz. size) *Campbell's® Chunky®* Split Pea with Ham Soup
1 cup low-fat milk
1 trip to The Super Salad Bar
1 teaspoon oil with unlimited vinegar as dressing
1 choice from The Fresh Fruit Stand

½ can (18¾ oz. size) *Campbell's® Chunky®* Turkey Soup
1 cup low-fat milk
1 trip to The Super Salad Bar
1 choice from The Fresh Fruit Stand

½ can (19 oz. size) *Campbell's® Chunky®* Old Fashioned Vegetable Beef Soup
1 cup low-fat milk

continued

Lunch

1	trip to The Super Salad Bar
1	teaspoon oil with unlimited vinegar as dressing
1	choice from The Fresh Fruit Stand

1	package (9½ oz. size) *Dining Lite*™ Chicken ala King
1	slice French bread
1	trip to The Super Salad Bar
1	choice from The Fresh Fruit Stand

1	package (8½ oz. size) *Dining Lite*™ Chicken Aloha
1	slice French bread
1	trip to The Super Salad Bar
1	tablespoon low-calorie dressing
1	choice from The Fresh Fruit Stand

1	package (11 oz.) *Dining Lite*™ Chicken Cacciatore
1	trip to The Super Salad Bar
1	tablespoon low-calorie dressing
1	choice from The Fresh Fruit Stand

1	package (12¾ oz. size) *Dining Lite*™ Chicken Vegetable Medley
1	slice whole wheat, rye or white bread
1	teaspoon margarine
1	trip to The Super Salad Bar
1	choice from The Fresh Fruit Stand

1	package (11 oz.) *Dining Lite*™ Seafood Vegetable Medley
1	cup low-fat milk
1	trip to The Super Salad Bar
1	teaspoon oil with unlimited vinegar as dressing
1	choice from The Fresh Fruit Stand

1	package (11 oz.) *Dining Lite*™ Zucchini Lasagna
1	trip to The Super Salad Bar
1	teaspoon oil with unlimited vinegar as dressing
1	choice from The Fresh Fruit Stand

The Menu Planner

Lunch

1 can (7½ oz. size) *Franco-American®* Beef Ravioli in Meat Sauce
1 cup low-fat milk
1 trip to The Super Salad Bar
1 choice from The Fresh Fruit Stand

---

1 can (7⅜ oz.) *Franco-American®* Spaghetti with Meatballs in Tomato Sauce
1 cup low-fat milk
1 trip to The Super Salad Bar
1 choice from The Fresh Fruit Stand

---

1 can (7½ oz. size) *Franco-American®* Spaghetti in Meat Sauce
1 cup low-fat milk
1 trip to The Super Salad Bar
1 choice from The Fresh Fruit Stand

---

1 cup *Friend's®* Small Pea Baked Beans
1 trip to the Super Salad Bar
1 choice from The Fresh Fruit Stand

---

1 package (10 oz.) *Green Giant®* Beef Chow Mein with Rice and Vegetables
1 trip to The Super Salad Bar
1 tablespoon low-calorie dressing
2 choices from The Fresh Fruit Stand

---

1 package (9 oz.) *Green Giant®* Beef Stew
1 slice French bread
1 trip to The Super Salad Bar
1 teaspoon oil with unlimited vinegar as dressing
1 choice from The Fresh Fruit Stand

---

1 package (9 oz.) *Green Giant®* Beef Stroganoff with Noodles
1 trip to The Super Salad Bar
1 choice from The Fresh Fruit Stand

---

1 package (9 oz.) *Green Giant®* Chicken Chow Mein with Rice and Vegetables

continued

The World's Most Convenient Diet

Lunch

1	trip to The Super Salad Bar
1	tablespoon low-calorie dressing
2	choices from The Fresh Fruit Stand

1	package (10 oz.) *Green Giant*® Chicken and Pea Pods in Sauce with Rice and Vegetables
1	trip to The Super Salad Bar
1	choice from The Fresh Fruit Stand

1	package (9 oz.) *Green Giant*® Lasagna
1	trip to The Super Salad Bar
1	teaspoon oil with unlimited vinegar as dressing
1	choice from The Fresh Fruit Stand

1	package (9 oz.) *Green Giant*® Macaroni and Cheese
1	trip to The Super Salad Bar
1	teaspoon oil with unlimited vinegar as dressing
1	choice from The Fresh Fruit Stand

1	package (10 oz.) *Green Giant*® Spaghetti with Meatballs with Tomato Sauce
1	choice from The Super Salad Bar

1	package (9 oz.) *Green Giant*® Steak and Green Peppers in Sauce with Rice and Vegetables
1	trip to The Super Salad Bar
1	teaspoon oil with unlimited vinegar as dressing
1	choice from The Fresh Fruit Stand

½	(10¾ oz. size) *La Pizzeria*™ Cheese Pizza
1	trip to The Super Salad Bar
1	choice from The Fresh Fruit Stand

2	*Mrs. Paul's*® Crispier Crunchier Fish Sticks on
1	sandwich bun
	topped with shredded lettuce, tomato slice
1	cup low-fat milk
1	choice from The Fresh Fruit Stand

1	*Pepperidge Farm*® Deli, Beef with Barbecue Sauce
1	trip to The Super Salad Bar

continued

The Menu Planner

Lunch

1	tablespoon low-calorie dressing
1	choice from The Fresh Fruit Stand

1	*Pepperidge Farm*® Deli, Sliced Beef with Brown Sauce
1	trip to The Super Salad Bar
2	choices from The Fresh Fruit Stand

1	*Pepperidge Farm*® Deli, Turkey, Ham and Cheese
1	trip to The Super Salad Bar
2	choices from The Fresh Fruit Stand

1	package (9 oz.) *Stouffer's*® Cheese Stuffed Pasta Shells with Meat Sauce
1	trip to The Super Salad Bar
1	teaspoon oil with unlimited vinegar as dressing
1	choice from The Fresh Fruit Stand

1	package (9½ oz. size) *Stouffer's*® Chicken a la King with Rice
1	trip to The Super Salad Bar
1	choice from The Fresh Fruit Stand

1	package (11¼ oz. size) *Stouffer's*® Chicken Cacciatore with Spaghetti
1	trip to The Super Salad Bar
1	choice from The Fresh Fruit Stand

1	package (8 oz.) *Stouffer's*® Chicken Chow Mein without Noodles
1	hard roll
1	teaspoon margarine
1	trip to The Super Salad Bar
1	choice from The Fresh Fruit Stand

1	package (8¾ oz.) *Stouffer's*® Chili Con Carne with Beans
1	slice French bread
1	trip to The Super Salad Bar
1	choice from The Fresh Fruit Stand

Lunch

1	package (8 oz.) *Stouffer's*® New England Clam Chowder Soup
1	cup low-fat milk
1	trip to The Super Salad Bar
1	choice from The Fresh Fruit Stand

1	package (10½ oz. size) *Stouffer's*® Single Serving Lasagna
1	trip to The Super Salad Bar
1	choice from The Fresh Fruit Stand

1	package (10½ oz. size) *Stouffer's*® Linguini with Clam Sauce
1	trip to The Super Salad Bar
1	choice from The Fresh Fruit Stand

½	package (12½ oz. size) *Stouffer's*® Cheese French Bread Pizza
½	cup low-fat milk
1	trip to The Super Salad Bar
1	choice from The Fresh Fruit Stand

1	package (8¼ oz. size) *Stouffer's*® Split Pea with Ham Soup
1	hard roll
1	teaspoon margarine
1	trip to The Super Salad Bar
1	choice from The Fresh Fruit Stand

1	package (9⅝ oz.) *Stouffer's*® *Lean Cuisine*® Beef and Pork Cannelloni with Mornay Sauce
1	hard roll
1	teaspoon margarine
1	trip to The Super Salad Bar
1	choice from The Fresh Fruit Stand

1	package (8⅝ oz.) *Stouffer's*® *Lean Cuisine*® Oriental Beef in Sauce with Vegetables and Rice
1	trip to The Super Salad Bar
1	teaspoon oil with unlimited vinegar as dressing
1	choice from The Fresh Fruit Stand

The Menu Planner

Lunch

- 1 package (9⅛ oz.) *Stouffer's® Lean Cuisine®* Cheese Cannelloni with Tomato Sauce
- 1 hard roll
- 1 trip to The Super Salad Bar
- 1 choice from The Fresh Fruit Stand

- 1 package (11¼ oz.) *Stouffer's® Lean Cuisine®* Chicken Chow Mein with Rice
- 1 slice French bread
- 1 trip to The Super Salad Bar
- 1 teaspoon oil with unlimited vinegar as dressing
- 1 choice from The Fresh Fruit Stand

- 1 package (8½ oz. size) *Stouffer's® Lean Cuisine®* Glazed Chicken with Vegetable Rice
- 1 hard roll
- 1 teaspoon margarine
- 1 trip to The Super Salad Bar
- 1 choice from The Fresh Fruit Stand

- 1 package (12¾ oz. size) *Stouffer's® Lean Cuisine®* Chicken and Vegetables with Vermicelli
- 1 trip to The Super Salad Bar
- 1 teaspoon oil with unlimited vinegar as dressing
- 1 choice from The Fresh Fruit Stand

- 1 package (12⅜ oz.) *Stouffer's® Lean Cuisine®* Filet of Fish Divan
- 1 slice of French bread
- 1 teaspoon margarine
- 1 trip to The Super Salad Bar
- 1 choice from The Fresh Fruit Stand

- 1 package (9 oz.) *Stouffer's® Lean Cuisine®* Filet of Fish Florentine
- 1 slice French bread
- 1 trip to The Super Salad Bar
- 1 tablespoon low-calorie dressing
- 1 choice from The Fresh Fruit Stand

- 1 package (10 oz.) *Stouffer's® Lean Cuisine®* Meatball Stew

continued

The World's Most Convenient Diet

Lunch

1	slice French bread
1	trip to The Super Salad Bar
1	teaspoon oil with unlimited vinegar
1	choice from The Fresh Fruit Stand

1	package (9½ oz. size) *Stouffer's® Lean Cuisine®* Salisbury Steak with Italian Style Sauce and Vegetables
1	hard roll
1	trip to The Super Salad Bar
1	choice from The Fresh Fruit Stand

1	package (11 oz.) *Stouffer's® Lean Cuisine®* Zucchini Lasagna
1	slice French bread
1	trip to The Super Salad Bar
1	choice from The Fresh Fruit Stand

1	package (290 grams) Swanson® *Le Menu*™ Chicken ála King
1	trip to The Super Salad Bar
1	choice from The Fresh Fruit Stand

1	package (326 grams) Swanson® *Le Menu*™ Pepper Steak
1	choice from The Fresh Fruit Stand

1	package (312 grams) Swanson® *Le Menu*™ Yankee Pot Roast
1	choice from The Fresh Fruit Stand

1	package (8 oz.) *Tabatchnick's®* Bean & Barley Soup
1	cup low-fat milk
1	hard roll
1	teaspoon margarine
1	trip to The Super Salad Bar
1	choice from The Fresh Fruit Stand

1	package (8 oz.) *Tabatchnick's®* Northern Bean Soup
1	cup low-fat milk
1	hard roll

continued

The Menu Planner

Lunch

1	teaspoon margarine
1	trip to The Super Salad Bar
1	choice from The Fresh Fruit Stand

1	package (8 oz.) *Tabatchnick's*® Lentil Soup
1	cup low-fat milk
6	soda crackers
1	trip to The Super Salad Bar
1	choice from The Fresh Fruit Stand

1	package (8 oz.) *Tabatchnick's*® Minestrone Soup
1	cup low-fat milk
6	soda crackers
1	trip to The Super Salad Bar
1	choice from The Fresh Fruit Stand

1	package (8 oz.) *Tabatchnick's*® Pea Soup
1	cup low-fat milk
6	soda crackers
1	trip to The Super Salad Bar
1	choice from The Fresh Fruit Stand

1	package (8 oz.) *Tabatchnick's*® Seafood Chowder
1	cup low-fat milk
6	soda crackers
1	trip to The Super Salad Bar
1	choice from The Fresh Fruit Stand

3	*Tyson*® *Chick'n Quick*® Chicken Sticks
1	sandwich bun
1	trip to The Super Salad Bar
1	choice from The Fresh Fruit Stand

1	serving (5 oz.) *Tyson*® *Chick'n Quick*® Cordon Bleu Chicken
1	trip to The Super Salad Bar
2	choices from The Fresh Fruit Stand

1	*Tyson*® *Turkey Quick*® Turkey Pattie
1	sandwich bun
1	trip to The Super Salad Bar

continued

Lunch

1	choice from The Fresh Fruit Stand

1	package (11 oz.) *Van De Kamp's*® Beef and Vegetables Szechwan with Rice
1	trip to The Super Salad Bar
1	choice from The Fresh Fruit Stand

½	package (12 oz. size) *Van De Kamp's*® Beef & Bean Burritos with Chili Salsa
1	trip to The Super Salad Bar
1	tablespoon low-calorie dressing
2	choices from The Fresh Fruit Stand

1	package (11 oz.) *Van De Kamp's*® Shredded Beef Enchiladas
1	trip to The Super Salad Bar
1	choice from The Fresh Fruit Stand

½	package (11¼ oz. size) *Van De Kamp's*® Chicken Enchilada Suiza
1	trip to The Super Salad Bar
1	tablespoon low-calorie dressing
2	choices from The Fresh Fruit Stand

1	package (8 oz.) *Wakefield*® Filet of Fish with Newburg Sauce
1	trip to The Super Salad Bar
1	tablespoon low-calorie dressing
2	choices from The Fresh Fruit Stand

1	package (6 oz.) *Wakefield*® Seafood Stuffed Potatoes
1	trip to The Super Salad Bar
1	tablespoon low-calorie dressing
2	choices from The Fresh Fruit Stand

1	package (8 oz.) *Wakefield*® Sole with Crab Stuffing and Lemon Sauce
1	hard roll
1	trip to The Super Salad Bar
1	choice from The Fresh Fruit Stand

The Menu Planner

Lunch

1	package (8 oz.) *Wakefield*® Sole Florentine with Mornay Sauce
1	trip to The Super Salad Bar
1	tablespoon low-calorie dressing
2	choices from The Fresh Fruit Stand

1	serving *Weaver*® Chicken Au Gratin
1	sandwich bun
1	trip to The Super Salad Bar
1	choice from The Fresh Fruit Stand

3	*Weaver*® Crispy Sticks
1	sandwich bun
1	trip to The Super Salad Bar
1	choice from The Fresh Fruit Stand

5	*Weaver*® Mini-Drums, Crispy or Herb 'n Spice Variety
1	sandwich bun
1	trip to The Super Salad Bar
1	choice from The Fresh Fruit Stand

1	*Weaver*® Rondelet; Original, Cheese or Italian Variety
1	sandwich bun
1	trip to The Super Salad Bar
1	choice from The Fresh Fruit Stand

Choice of   **When You're The Cook**

1	Chef's salad made with
3	ounces of any type lean meat, cut in strips and variety of salad vegetables from The Super Salad Bar
1	tablespoon low-calorie dressing
1	hard roll or slice French bread
2	choices from The Fresh Fruit Stand

½	cup cottage cheese on a lettuce leaf served with
2	choices from The Fresh Fruit Stand
1	granola bar, any variety

The World's Most Convenient Diet

Lunch

3	ounces sliced lean beef served on
2	slices whole wheat, rye or white bread top with extras from The Super Salad Bar
2	choices from The Fresh Fruit Stand

3	ounces sliced chicken or turkey served on
2	slices whole wheat, rye or white bread top with extras from The Super Salad Bar
2	choices from The Fresh Fruit Stand

3	ounces broiled, baked or poached fish served with lemon
1	slice whole wheat, rye or white bread
1	trip to The Super Salad Bar
1	tablespoon low-calorie dressing
1	choice from The Fresh Fruit Stand

1	(3 oz.) broiled lean hamburger served open face on
1	slice whole wheat, rye or white bread top with extras from The Super Salad Bar
1	trip to The Super Salad Bar
1	tablespoon low-calorie dressing
1	choice from The Fresh Fruit Stand

3	ounces lean meat or poultry, broiled or baked
1	cup cooked vegetables from The Super Salad Bar
1	slice whole wheat, rye or white bread
1	teaspoon margarine
1	choice from The Fresh Fruit Stand

Dinner

83	Fast Food Fare
84	Heat and Eat
93	Cool and Quick
94	Home Cooking

The Menu Planner

Dinner

Choice of	**Fast Food Fare**

Remember to be accurate when ordering these items. Be specific and don't add extra sauces. Bring your fresh fruit from home.

1	*Arby's*® French Dip
2	choices from The Fresh Fruit Stand

1	*Arby's*® Regular Roast Beef Sandwich (no sauce)
2	choices from The Fresh Fruit Stand

1	*Dairy Queen Brazier*® Single Hamburger with Cheese
1	choice from The Fresh Fruit Stand

1	*McDonald's*® *Quarter Pounder*® (no cheese)
1	choice from The Fresh Fruit Stand

2	*Taco Bell*® *Bellbeefers*®
1	choice from The Fresh Fruit Stand

2	*Taco Bell*® Tacos
2	choices from The Fresh Fruit Stand

1	*Wendy's*® Chicken Sandwich top with lettuce and tomato
1	trip to The Super Salad Bar
1	tablespoon low-calorie dressing
1	choice from The Fresh Fruit Stand

1	*Wendy's*® Chicken Sandwich with Cheese
1	choice from The Fresh Fruit Stand

1	8-ounce serving *Wendy's*® Chili
1	trip to the Super Salad Bar
1	tablespoon low-calorie dressing
1	choice from The Fresh Fruit Stand

1	*Wendy's*® Taco Salad
1	choice from The Fresh Fruit Stand

The World's Most Convenient Diet

Dinner

Choice of	Heat And Eat
1	package (11¼ oz.) *Armour Classic Lite*™ Chicken Burgundy
1	slice whole wheat, rye or white bread
1	trip to The Super Salad Bar
1	teaspoon oil with unlimited vinegar as dressing
1	choice from The Fresh Fruit Stand
1	package (10 oz.) *Armour Classic Lite*™ Chicken Oriental
1	slice whole wheat, rye or white bread
1	teaspoon margarine
1	trip to The Super Salad Bar
1	tablespoon low-calorie dressing
1	choice from The Fresh Fruit Stand
1	package(13¼ oz.) *Armour Classic Lite*™ Filet of Cod Divan
1	slice whole wheat, rye or white bread
1	teaspoon margarine
1	trip to The Super Salad Bar
1	teaspoon oil with unlimited vinegar as dressing
1	choice from The Fresh Fruit Stand
1	package (10 oz.) *Armour Classic Lite*™ Turf and Surf
1	slice whole wheat, rye or white bread
1	teaspoon margarine
1	trip to The Super Salad Bar
1	tablespoon low-calorie dressing
1	choice from The Fresh Fruit Stand
1	package (11 oz.) *Armour Classic Lite*™ Turkey Parmesan
1	slice whole wheat, rye or white bread
1	teaspoon margarine
1	trip to The Super Salad Bar
1	teaspoon oil with unlimited vinegar as dressing
1	choice from The Fresh Fruit Stand

The Menu Planner

Dinner

- 1 package (11 oz.) *Armour Classic Lite™* Veal Pepper Steak
- 1 slice whole wheat, rye or white bread
- 1 teaspoon margarine
- 1 trip to The Super Salad Bar
- 1 tablespoon low-calorie dressing
- 1 choice from The Fresh Fruit Stand

- 1 package (10½ oz.) *Armour Dinner Classic®* Beef Burgundy
- 1 slice whole wheat, rye or white bread
- 1 teaspoon margarine
- 1 choice from The Fresh Fruit Stand

- 1 package (11¼ oz.) *Armour Dinner Classic®* Beef Stroganoff
- 1 trip to The Super Salad Bar
- 1 teaspoon oil with unlimited vinegar as dressing
- 1 choice from The Fresh Fruit Stand

- 1 package (11¾ oz.) *Armour Dinner Classic®* Chicken Fricassee
- 1 trip to The Super Salad Bar
- 1 teaspoon oil with unlimited vinegar as dressing
- 1 choice from The Fresh Fruit Stand

- 1 package (12 oz.) *Armour Dinner Classic®* Cod Almondine
- 1 slice whole wheat, rye or white bread
- 1 teaspoon margarine
- 1 choice from The Fresh Fruit Stand

- 1 package (11 oz.) *Armour Dinner Classic®* Sirloin Tips
- 1 slice whole wheat, rye or white bread
- 1 teaspoon margarine
- 1 choice from The Fresh Fruit Stand

- 1 package (10 oz.) *Armour Dinner Classic®* Teriyaki Steak
- 1 trip to The Super Salad Bar

continued

The World's Most Convenient Diet

Dinner

1	teaspoon oil with unlimited vinegar as dressing
1	choice from The Fresh Fruit Stand

1	cup *B&M*® Red Kidney, Small Pea or Yellow Eye Baked Beans
1	cup low-fat milk
1	trip to The Super Salad Bar
1	choice from The Fresh Fruit Stand

1	package (10 oz.) *Banquet*® Beef with Gravy Dinner
1	slice whole wheat, rye or white bread
1	trip to The Super Salad Bar
1	choice from The Fresh Fruit Stand

½	can (19½ oz. size) *Campbell's*® *Chunky*® Chili Beef Soup
1	cup low-fat milk
1	trip to The Super Salad Bar
1	teaspoon oil with unlimited vinegar as dressing
1	choice from The Fresh Fruit Stand

1	package (9½ oz.) *Dining Lite*™ Chicken à la King
1	cup low-fat milk
1	slice French bread
1	trip to The Super Salad Bar
1	choice from The Fresh Fruit Stand

1	package (8½ oz.) *Dining Lite*™ Chicken Aloha
1	slice whole wheat, rye or white bread
1	teaspoon margarine
1	trip to The Super Salad Bar
1	tablespoon low-calorie dressing
2	choices from The Fresh Fruit Stand

1	package (11 oz.) *Dining Lite*™ Chicken Cacciatore
1	slice whole wheat, rye or white bread
1	teaspoon margarine
1	trip to The Super Salad Bar
1	teaspoon oil with unlimited vinegar as dressing
1	choice from The Fresh Fruit Stand

The Menu Planner

Dinner

- 1 package (12¾ oz.) *Dining Lite*™ Chicken Vegetable Medley
- 1 cup low-fat milk
- 1 slice whole wheat, rye or white bread
- 1 teaspoon margarine
- 1 choice from The Fresh Fruit Stand

- 1 package (11 oz.) *Dining Lite*™ Zucchini Lasagna
- 1 cup low-fat milk
- 1 trip to The Super Salad Bar
- 1 teaspoon oil with unlimited vinegar as dressing
- 1 choice from The Fresh Fruit Stand

- 1 package (9 oz.) *Green Giant*® Beef Stew
- 1 cup low-fat milk
- 1 slice French bread
- 1 trip to The Super Salad Bar
- 1 teaspoon oil with unlimited vinegar as dressing
- 1 choice from The Fresh Fruit Stand

- 1 package (9 oz.) *Green Giant*® Beef Stroganoff with noodles
- 1 cup milk
- 1 trip to The Super Salad Bar
- 1 choice from The Fresh Fruit Stand

- 1 package (10 oz.) *Green Giant*® Chicken and Broccoli with Rice in Cheese Sauce
- 1 slice French bread
- 1 trip to The Super Salad Bar
- 1 choice from The Fresh Fruit Stand

- 1 package (10 oz.) *Green Giant*® Chicken with Pea Pods in Sauce with Rice and Vegetables
- 1 cup low-fat milk
- 1 trip to The Super Salad Bar
- 1 choice from The Fresh Fruit Stand

- 1 package (9 oz.) *Green Giant*® Lasagna
- 1 cup low-fat milk
- 1 trip to The Super Salad Bar

continued

Dinner

1	teaspoon oil with unlimited vinegar as dressing
1	choice from The Fresh Fruit Stand

1	package (9 oz.) *Green Giant*® Steak and Green Peppers in Sauce with Rice and Vegetables
1	trip to The Super Salad Bar
1	teaspoon oil with unlimited vinegar as dressing
1	choice from The Fresh Fruit Stand

1	fillet (6 oz.) *Mrs. Paul's*® Light and Natural Cod Fillets
1	slice French bread
1	trip to The Super Salad Bar
1	tablespoon low-calorie dressing
2	choices from The Fresh Fruit Stand

1	fillet (6 oz.) *Mrs. Paul's*® Light and Natural Flounder Fillets
1	slice French bread
1	trip to The Super Salad Bar
1	tablespoon low-calorie dressing
2	choices from The Fresh Fruit Stand

1	fillet (6 oz.) *Mrs. Paul's*® Light and Natural Sole Fillets
1	slice French bread
1	trip to The Super Salad Bar
1	tablespoon low-calorie dressing
2	choices from The Fresh Fruit Stand

1	package (9½ oz.) *Stouffer's*® Chicken á la King with Rice
½	cup low-fat milk
1	trip to The Super Salad Bar
1	tablespoon low-calorie dressing
1	choice from The Fresh Fruit Stand

1	package (11¼ oz.) *Stouffer's*® Chicken Cacciatore with Spaghetti
1	slice French bread
1	trip to The Super Salad Bar

continued

The Menu Planner

Dinner

1	teaspoon oil with unlimited vinegar as dressing
1	choice from The Fresh Fruit Stand

1	package (10½ oz.) *Stouffer's*® Single Serving Lasagna
1	trip to The Super Salad Bar
1	teaspoon oil with unlimited vinegar as dressing
1	choice from The Fresh Fruit Stand

1	package (10¼ oz.) *Stouffer's*® Scallops & Shrimp Mariner with Rice
1	trip to The Super Salad Bar
2	choices from The Fresh Fruit Stand

1	package (8¼ oz.) *Stouffer's*® Split Pea with Ham Soup
1	cup low-fat milk
1	hard roll
1	teaspoon margarine
1	choice from The Fresh Fruit Stand

1	package (9⅝ oz.) *Stouffer's*® Lean Cuisine® Beef and Pork Cannelloni with Mornay Sauce
1	slice whole wheat, rye or white bread
1	teaspoon margarine
1	trip to The Super Salad Bar
1	teaspoon oil with unlimited vinegar as dressing
2	choices from The Fresh Fruit Stand

1	package (9⅛ oz.) *Stouffer's*® Lean Cuisine® Cheese Cannelloni with Tomato Sauce
1	slice French bread
1	trip to The Super Salad Bar
1	tablespoon low-calorie dressing
2	choices from The Fresh Fruit Stand

1	package (8½ oz.) *Stouffer's*® Lean Cuisine® Glazed Chicken with Vegetable Rice
1	slice whole wheat, rye or white bread
1	teaspoon margarine
1	trip to The Super Salad Bar

continued

The World's Most Convenient Diet

Dinner

1	tablespoon low-calorie dressing
1	choice from The Fresh Fruit Stand

1	package (12⅜ oz.) *Stouffer's® Lean Cuisine®* Filet of Fish Divan
1	slice whole wheat, rye or white bread
1	teaspoon margarine
1	trip to The Super Salad Bar
1	tablespoon low-calorie dressing
1	choice from The Fresh Fruit Stand

1	package (9 oz.) *Stouffer's® Lean Cuisine®* Filet of Fish Florentine
1	slice whole wheat, rye or white bread
1	teaspoon margarine
1	trip to The Super Salad Bar
1	tablespoon low-calorie dressing
2	choices from The Fresh Fruit Stand

1	package (9½ oz.) *Stouffer's® Lean Cuisine®* Salisbury Steak with Italian Style Sauce and Vegetables
1	slice French bread
1	trip to The Super Salad Bar
1	tablespoon low-calorie dressing
2	choices from The Fresh Fruit Stand

1	package (11 oz.) *Stouffer's® Lean Cuisine®* Zucchini Lasagna
1	slice whole wheat, rye or white bread
1	teaspoon margarine
1	trip to The Super Salad Bar
1	teaspoon oil with unlimited vinegar as dressing
2	choices from The Fresh Fruit Stand

1	package (326 grams) Swanson® *Le Menu*™ Beef Sirloin Tips
1	trip to The Super Salad Bar
2	choices from The Fresh Fruit Stand

1	package (290 grams) Swanson® *Le Menu*™ Chicken á la King

continued

The Menu Planner

Dinner

1 slice French bread
1 trip to The Super Salad Bar
1 teaspoon oil with unlimited vinegar as dressing
1 choice from The Fresh Fruit Stand

---

1 package (326 grams) *Swanson® Le Menu*™ Breast of Chicken Parmigiana
1 trip to The Super Salad Bar
1 choice from The Fresh Fruit Stand

---

1 package (326 grams) *Swanson® Le Menu*™ Pepper Steak
1 trip to The Super Salad Bar
1 tablespoon low-calorie dressing
1 choice from The Fresh Fruit Stand

---

1 package (312 grams) *Swanson® Le Menu*™ Yankee Pot Roast
1 trip to The Super Salad Bar
1 tablespoon low-calorie dressing
1 choice from The Fresh Fruit Stand

---

1 serving (5 oz.) *Tyson® Chick 'n Quick®* Cordon Bleu Chicken
1 slice French bread
1 trip to The Super Salad Bar
1 tablespoon low-calorie dressing
1 choice from The Fresh Fruit Stand

---

1 package (11 oz.) *Van De Kamp's®* Beef Chow Mein Mandarin
1 trip to The Super Salad Bar
2 choices from The Fresh Fruit Stand

---

1 package (11 oz.) *Van De Kamp's®* Beef and Vegetables Szechwan with Rice
1 cup low-fat milk
1 trip to The Super Salad Bar
1 choice from The Fresh Fruit Stand

Dinner

1	package (11 oz.) *Van De Kamp's*® Shredded Beef Enchiladas
1	trip to The Super Salad Bar
1	tablespoon low-calorie dressing
2	choices from The Fresh Fruit Stand

1	package (11 oz.) *Van De Kamp's*® Almond Chicken Cantonese with Rice
1	trip to The Super Salad Bar
1	choice from The Fresh Fruit Stand

1	package (11 oz.) *Van De Kamp's*® Chicken Chow Mein Mandarin
1	trip to The Super Salad Bar
2	choices from The Fresh Fruit Stand

1	package (11 oz.) *Van De Kamp's*® Creamy Spinach Lasagna
1	trip to The Super Salad Bar
2	choices from The Fresh Fruit Stand

1	package (8 oz.) *Wakefield*® Filet of Fish with Newburg Sauce
1	slice French bread
1	teaspoon margarine
1	trip to The Super Salad Bar
1	tablespoon low-calorie dressing
2	choices from The Fresh Fruit Stand

1	package (8 oz.) *Wakefield*® Sole with Crab Stuffing and Lemon Sauce
1	slice French bread
1	trip to The Super Salad Bar
1	tablespoon low-calorie dressing
1	choice from The Fresh Fruit Stand

1	package (8 oz.) *Wakefield*® Sole Florentine with Mornay Sauce
1	slice French bread
1	trip to The Super Salad Bar
1	teaspoon oil with unlimited vinegar as dressing
2	choices from The Fresh Fruit Stand

The Menu Planner

Dinner

1	serving *Weaver®* Chicken Au Gratin
1	sandwich bun
1	cup low-fat milk
1	trip to The Super Salad Bar
1	choice from The Fresh Fruit Stand

3	*Weaver®* Crispy Sticks
1	sandwich bun
1	cup low-fat milk
1	trip to The Super Salad Bar
1	choice from The Fresh Fruit Stand

1	*Weaver®* Rondelet; Original, Cheese or Italian variety
1	sandwich bun
1	cup low-fat milk
1	trip to The Super Salad Bar
1	choice from The Fresh Fruit Stand

Choice of   Cool & Quick

2	slices *Eckrich® Calorie Watcher™* Slender Sliced Corned Beef top with extras from The Super Salad Bar
2	slices whole wheat, rye or white bread
1	cup low-fat milk
1	trip to The Super Salad Bar
1	teaspoon oil with unlimited vinegar as dressing
1	choice from The Fresh Fruit Stand

1	Julienne Salad made with
2	slices *Eckrich® Calorie Watcher™* Sliced Cooked Ham and
1	sliced hard-cooked egg and unlimited vegetables from The Super Salad Bar
1	teaspoon oil with unlimited vinegar as dressing
1	cup low-fat milk
1	hard roll or slice French bread
1	choice from The Fresh Fruit Stand

3	slices *Louis Rich™* Oven Roasted Turkey Breast

continued

The World's Most Convenient Diet

Dinner

2	slices whole wheat, rye or white bread top with extras from The Super Salad Bar
1	cup low-fat milk
1	trip to The Super Salad Bar
1	tablespoon low-calorie dressing
1	choice from The Fresh Fruit Stand

2	slices *Oscar Mayer*® 93% Fat-free Canadian Style Bacon
2	slices whole wheat, rye or white bread top with extras from The Super Salad Bar
1	cup low-fat milk
1	trip to The Super Salad Bar
1	teaspoon oil with unlimited vinegar as dressing
1	choice from The Fresh Fruit Stand

½	can (6 or 7 oz. size) water packed Tuna, any brand including *Bumble Bee*®, *Chicken of the Sea*® or *Star-Kist*®, mixed with
1	tablespoon mayonnaise or salad dressing, chopped onion, celery and green pepper
2	slices whole wheat, rye or white bread
2	choices from The Fresh Fruit Stand

¾	cup cottage cheese, any brand
4	soda crackers
1	trip to The Super Salad Bar
1	tablespoon low-calorie dressing
2	choices from The Fresh Fruit Stand

Choice of   **Home Cooking**

4	ounces baked or broiled lean beef
½	cup potatoes, rice or noodles
1	cup cooked vegetable selected from The Super Salad Bar List
1	teaspoon margarine
1	choice from The Fresh Fruit Stand

1	grilled cheese sandwich made with
2	ounces non-processed cheese including Swiss, Cheddar, Muenster or Monterey Jack

continued

The Menu Planner

Dinner

2	slices whole wheat, rye or white bread
1	teaspoon margarine
1	trip to The Super Salad Bar
1	tablespoon low-calorie dressing
1	choice from The Fresh Fruit Stand

4	ounces baked or broiled chicken with skin removed
½	cup potatoes, rice or noodles
3	teaspoons margarine allowed in preparation
1	trip to The Super Salad Bar
1	tablespoon low-calorie dressing
1	choice from The Fresh Fruit Stand

4	ounces broiled or grilled barbecued chicken, skin removed
2	tablespoons barbecue sauce
1	hard roll or slice French bread
1	teaspoon margarine
1	trip to The Super Salad Bar
1	tablespoon low-calorie dressing
1	choice from The Fresh Fruit Stand

4	ounces broiled lean hamburger served on
1	hamburger roll
	top with extras from The Super Salad Bar
1	trip to The Super Salad Bar
1	tablespoon low-calorie dressing
1	choice from The Fresh Fruit Stand

1	Pasta dinner made with
3	ounces lean ground beef added to
½	cup tomato sauce
1	cup cooked pasta
1	trip to The Super Salad Bar
1	tablespoon low-calorie dressing
1	choice from The Fresh Fruit Stand

4	ounces baked, broiled or grilled seafood served with lemon
1	small baked potato served with
2	teaspoons margarine

continued

The World's Most Convenient Diet

Dinner

1	trip to The Super Salad Bar
1	tablespoon low-calorie dressing
1	choice from The Fresh Fruit Stand

1	(4 oz.) baked or broiled pork, lean portion
½	cup potatoes, rice or noodles
1	cup cooked vegetable selected from The Super Salad Bar list
1	teaspoon margarine
1	choice from The Fresh Fruit Stand

4	ounces roast turkey, skin removed
1	small baked sweet potato
1	teaspoon margarine
1	cup cooked vegetable selected from The Super Salad Bar list
1	choice from The Fresh Fruit Stand

1	(4 oz.) baked or broiled veal or lamb chop, lean portion
1	small baked potato
1	cup cooked vegetable selected from The Super Salad Bar list
2	teaspoons margarine
1	choice from The Fresh Fruit Stand

Chapter Six
Recommended Multivitamin-With-Minerals Supplements

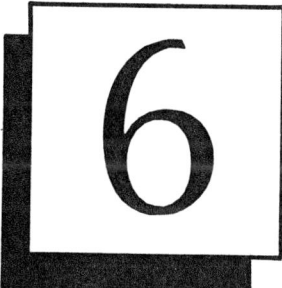

Recommended Multivitamin-With-Minerals Supplements

Adequate supplies of vitamins and minerals are essential to good health. We obtain these nutrients from the food we eat. No single food is nutritionally complete by itself; a proper combination of foods makes up a balanced diet.

With this in mind, *The World's Most Convenient Diet* has been designed to provide maximum nutrition along with ease in preparation. We do recommend a daily vitamin-with-minerals supplement, however, to help ensure adequate intake of calcium and iron. It is not uncommon to see less than recommended levels of these two nutrients consumed in weight-reduction diets as well as in the typical American diet.

The following chart lists some non-prescription multi-vitamin-with-minerals preparations. The brands contain nonexcessive amounts of nutrients, providing 50 to 100 percent of the Recommended Dietary Allowance[1] for iron and a range of 12 to 25 percent of the RDA for calcium. Additional calcium can be received from the milk and daily products included in the diet plan.

This is not meant to be a complete list; you may even find a generic equivalent. Remember not to exceed Recommended Daily Allowance levels (found on the label) by more than 200 percent if selecting your own supplement. High doses of vitamins and minerals are unnecessary and are potentially toxic.

Brand	Company
Gevral® Tablets	Lederle
Hypomins™	Pasadena Research
Minro-Plex Capsules™	Mallard
Min-Viteral Capsules™	Kay Pharmaceuticals
One-A-Day® Plus Minerals Tablets	Miles Labs
Stuart Formula® Tablets	Stuart
Vitagetts Tablets™	Vortech Pharmaceuticals

---

[1] Recommended Dietary Allowances. Revised 1980. Food and Nutrition Board, National Academy of Sciences – National Research Council.

Chapter Seven
Taking You Through Thick to Thin

103   Determining a Target Weight

104   Developing a New Approach to Eating

105   Seven Techniques to Alter Your Eating Habits

106   Your Eating Signals: What are They?

107   Fitness vs. Fat

**Taking You Through
Thick To Thin**

Now that you've been introduced to *The World's Most Convenient Diet*, you can see how simple the mechanics of losing weight can be. Not only has the nutrient counting been done for you, but so has the cooking. What you need to do now is make a promise to *yourself*. Notice, please, the promise is up to you. If your reason for dieting is not because you want to lose weight, there's a problem. You should not be dieting because a friend or relative said you should be. What happens when they're not around? And don't diet for a reward. You can easily convince yourself the reward isn't important. As far as the buddy system goes, well, it's a great idea for swimming, but if your buddy quits the diet, he's apt to pull you down, too! This must be your own personal commitment. The will power will then come from you. Since it's not dependent on an outside force, it will always be available. In this chapter, we will get you started thinking and acting successfully about your diet. In fact, we're going to take you through thick to thin.

Determining Target Weight

The best place to begin is by defining your target weight. This isn't difficult. We suggest using the following method.

First, determine your height without shoes. Don't just guess; have someone help you do it accurately. If you have access to a measuring rod like the one attached to a doctor's scale, use that. Stand erect with your shoulders squared and have the crossbar rest gently on your head. If you don't have the use of a scale with a measuring rod, stand against a wall, assuming the same correct posture. Have someone mark your height on the wall and then measure from the mark to the floor. Now use the following formula to find your desired body weight.

Women: Allow 100 pounds for the first five feet of height. Then add five pounds for each inch over five feet.

Men: Allow 106 pounds for the first five feet of height. Then add six pounds for each inch over five feet.

For example, if you are a woman who is five-foot-five, your target weight should be 100 pounds + 25 pounds = 125 pounds. A man who is six-foot-two should have a target weight of 106 pounds + 84 pounds = 190 pounds.

These formulas are for medium-built body frames. If you have a small frame, you need only to lose an additional five to 10 pounds. Conversely, if you have a large body frame, allow yourself to carry an additional 10 to 15 pounds.

Now that you've defined the challenge of how much weight to lose, minimize it. Smaller challenges are not as formidable. If you are faced with losing 40 pounds after calculating your target weight, you may become overwhelmed. Don't let this happen. Get a calendar and set a first week goal of a three-pound weight loss. Anything more than this is a bonus. The following week, promise yourself a two-pound loss. Be realistic. A goal for the first month on *The World's Most Convenient Diet* should be approximately 9 to 11 pounds. After that, two pounds a week is an anticipated rate. Weigh yourself once a week, preferably at the same time of day. Mark your calendar accordingly. By using a short-term achievement plan, your 40-pound challenge is not nearly as great. You have also given yourself a chance to be successful each week.

Along with marking your goals on the calendar, jot down encouraging notes to yourself on certain days. If, for example, you notice that an evening at a friend's home is scheduled for later in the week, there should be some "you-can-do-it" notes a couple of days in advance. Any message that has a special meaning for you will work. Forewarned is forearmed!

Developing A New Approach To Eating

There is always an excitement that accompanies the beginning of a diet. You are filled with high hopes, great expectations and motivation. Sustaining those feelings is important and is going to take some will power. Be aware of your goals – both short and long term. To achieve them, you will need to be changing *what* you eat, *how* you eat and *why* you eat. *The World's Most Convenient Diet* has incorporated the change in *what* you eat. By choosing your day's food from the extensive menu planning section, you are participating in a type of forecasting. It is a very effective technique. Studies have demonstrated that you are less apt to stray from a diet if you have forecasted a day's (or week's) eating activity. We encourage you to make a weekly shopping list so that your kitchen will be stocked with exactly the items you are allowed. To make this technique more familiar to you, the sample seven-day diet plan is accompanied by a shopping list. Remember, planning ahead is not difficult. Once each week you will need to choose meals for seven days from the menu planning section. Compile the list, go to the supermarket and you are done. There's no reason why shopping for two or three weeks at a time wouldn't work. Do whatever is best for you.

Taking You Through Thick To Thin

Seven Techniques To Alter Your Eating Habits

Don't be fooled! Simply changing what you eat is not the only important ingredient to losing weight. *How* you eat is also crucial. In taking you through thick to thin, we suggest these rules when meal time comes around:

1. **Check the menu you selected.** Gather the entree, salad, fruit, beverage and whatever else is specified. While preparing the main course (this will be easy!), allow yourself to imagine how much you are going to enjoy the meal.
2. **Be seated at a table when you eat.** Do not start eating until your entire meal is set before you. Think of standing and eating as incompatible behavior. It should remind you of trying to pat your head while rubbing your stomach. We know of some dieters who have gone so far as to have a designated seat and will not allow themselves to eat unless they were in that chair. The value of this idea is obvious. Once into the habit of associating eating with a certain spot, you are unlikely to munch in other areas, such as the living room, family room, office or car. So, if you'd like, become a "designated sitter."
3. **Set down your eating utensils between mouthfuls.** Do not attempt to fill your fork or spoon with the next bite until you have swallowed the previous bite. This is a suggestion we've all heard before. (It usually goes hand-in-hand with chewing a mouthful 39 times or so before swallowing!) It *is* amazing, though, to watch how many people have their fork ready and waiting for their next bite before they've even enjoyed the previous one. Observe some fellow diners the next chance you get.
4. **Chew each mouthful slowly.** Speaking of 39 times! We don't think it's fun or necessary to pick a number of times to chew a mouthful (consider the dilemma of mashed potatoes versus sirloin tips!), but do learn to eat slower.
5. **Plan a five-minute break in each meal.** This could be a few minutes of clearing the table between your entree and dessert or perhaps before your cup of coffee. One dieter found this break was the ideal way of ensuring the dinner dishes got done. It's nice to enjoy a cup of coffee without the clutter of dirty dishes.
6. **Develop a "20-minute clock."** Try to have a meal last for that length of time. (This may pose a problem at breakfast, but should be feasible for lunch and dinner.) When you are eating three meals a day, it is important that you make the occasion last longer than five or 10 minutes. Otherwise, you are often left feeling unsatisfied.
7. **When the meal is done, allow yourself to realize how much you enjoyed it.** Also enjoy the "non-stuffed" feeling you will have eating an appropriately sized meal. You'll feel great about yourself!

These are seven behavior changing and awareness techniques to help alter how you eat. You can be your own personal consultant and come up with other ideas. For example, one woman decided to eat restaurant-style. She began each meal with a glass of ice water with a lemon twist. The salad came next. The entree was followed by fruit or dessert. However, before the last course, the table was cleared and the coffee freshly brewed.

Another suggestion is to establish a time when the meal will begin. You might choose to come home from work and relax for half an hour before you even begin preparing the meal. You'll have the extra time to relax because of the minimal preparation time on this diet. The advantange of waiting is that eating will not be a hurried event, but rather something to anticipate and enjoy. Some dieters who are not working outside the home find the couple of hours just before dinner to be a pretty tough test. This is a great opportunity to do some busy work around the house. (Not in the kitchen, please!) Sitting down to read or watch television just might do you in during this time.

Your Eating Signals: What Are They?

By now you may be wondering if eating will ever again be an uncomplicated event! Yes, it will be, but it is important to become aware of how and why you eat. Otherwise, how do you prevent yourself from lapsing into bad habits? Some veteran dieters recognize this "lapsing into bad habits" as the urge to cheat. The first couple of weeks on most diets are fairly smooth, probably because of the diet's novelty and the fact that weight loss during the first two weeks is usually greater than the following losses per week. But after the third week or so, dieters often feel the urge to "cheat." Learning to cope with this is your key to successful weight loss. You must become aware of *why* you want to eat.

It's amazing how many different reasons exist for eating. Hunger, anxiety, boredom, depression, excitement, happiness or sadness are just part of the extensive list of eating cues. Consider this example: Every afternoon, when you were school age, you would come home after classes and have a snack. Can you see how after 12 years, just the mere fact of coming home and walking into a kitchen is a signal to eat? Of course!

Let's do some self-awareness work. We had one dieter who had difficulty coping with a chronic case of boredom on Sunday afternoons. Any diet that started on a Monday morning usually ended the following Sunday with a binge. Monday through Friday was a breeze. Saturday was a fairly busy day, but Sundays just afforded too much time to think about eating. And eating won out. When this woman objectively looked at her solution to boredom – eating – she

Taking You Through Thick To Thin

saw it was an illogical response. When you are bored, find an activity that is interesting and stimulating for you. Is walking into the kitchen and raiding the cupboards and refrigerator that exciting?

The question that you must stop to ask yourself (you may even have to yell so you'll listen) is: "Why do I want to eat this?" Have a conversation. "Is it because I am angry?" "Is it because I am sad?" Look at matters clearly. If you are sad, look for something to cheer you. You know that adding extra calories and extra inches will only make you sadder. If you are anxious about something, sit down and analyze the problem. There's a good chance you wouldn't list eating as a solution to the problem.

Sometimes it is not an emotional signal that makes you want to eat. Instead, it's a physical cue. The aroma from the bakery as you walk past, the sight of food on a television commercial – we are all aware of how powerful these signals can be. The next time you are tempted to eat food that is not planned in your daily diet, ask yourself why. If the answer is that some emotion is causing that feeling, deal with the emotion in an appropriate manner. If some physical cue has triggered the urge to eat, tell yourself that it is not part of your plan. Put yourself in control of the situation.

If you feel hungry just prior to a meal, tell yourself this is only appropriate on a weight-loss diet. View it as a good sign, a symptom of success. Think about it! Feeling extremely full after a large meal or an eating binge never makes you feel as though you are getting thinner. On the other hand, a few hunger pangs indicate that you are making progress toward your weekly goal. Be encouraged by your growling stomach!

Fitness Vs. Fat

Exercise is very important in your quest for a healthy weight. We think it's just as beneficial for reaching your desired weight as is our diet plan. Not only can exercise help use up some extra calories and tone your muscles, it can also help you feel good by reducing emotional stress and tension. And it offers a built-in reward system. Remember how wonderful you felt about yourself the last time you did 30 sit-ups or rode your exercise bike for half an hour? There's no guilt at all associated with exercising – only a feeling of accomplishment. And physically fit people look great!

There are two things you need to do when choosing an exercise program. First, consult a physician if you have not had a physical examination in the last year. Find out what your doctor considers an appropriate level of exertion.

Second, shop around for the activity that would be best for you.

Your goal should be an exercise you would do at least three times a week. Consider a few factors here. How much time do you realistically have to devote to a physical activity program? How flexible is your lifestyle? Do you prefer a sport that offers a scheduled time, such as league play or an exercise class, or do you prefer an activity that can be done at your leisure? Would you be more likely to stick to a program if you could do it at home, such as riding an exercise bike? Or would you prefer a combination of activities? You can choose a program you do by yourself or opt for a more competitive sport in which you have an opponent. By the way, here's a word of caution on exercising (or dieting) the buddy-system way: Be stronger than your partner. Your buddy could tire of the whole regime and try to drag you down. Don't be sabotaged! Choose a program you're going to like and stick to it!

What are your options? Exercise falls into two categories: aerobic and non-aerobic. Aerobic exercises place a significant demand on the body for oxygen, which calls upon your fat deposits to deliver the energy. So on a regular aerobic program, your fat deposits will be reduced. In addition, your heart and lungs will become stronger. Aerobic activities characteristically:

1. are done continuously for a minimum of 12 to 15 minutes;
2. are performed strenuously enough to place a significant demand on the cardiovascular system.

Swimming, jogging, dancing, brisk walking and cycling are examples of aerobic activities. Cross-country skiing and swimming top the list as excellent workouts. Check your library for resource books on this type of exercise. Your local YMCA/YWCA or adult education classes may have aerobic programs.

Non-aerobic exercises do not demand as much oxygen as aerobic activities. Your body burns its readily available carbohydrate supply to provide the energy for this type of exercise. Non-aerobic programs do offer increased muscle strength, muscle tone and flexibility, which is beneficial while losing weight. Think of how good your arm and stomach muscles feel when they're in shape! A home exercise program that includes sit-ups, leg lifts and waist bends are examples of non-aerobic exercises. Tennis, body building and slower-paced walking are others. Again, check your library, local Y or adult education courses for good programs.

It should be clear by now that the person taking you through thick to thin is none other than yourself. Begin with a commitment to this weight-loss program. Determine your goals and mark them clearly on your calendar. The diet plan itself is simple. *You* must take charge of assessing your eating habits and then change the ones that prevent you from eating in a healthy, controlled manner. Embark on a well-planned physical fitness program. You'll enjoy the only remaining tasks: Applauding yourself and keeping track of the pounds you lose!

Chapter Eight
Nutrients

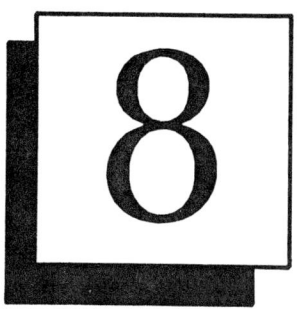

111 Protein
112 Fat
113 Carbohydrates
114 Fluids and Electrolytes
114 Fiber
115 Vitamins and Minerals

Nutrients

When most people go on diets, they immediately think of calories. "How many calories must I eliminate to lose weight?" "How many calories can I consume and still become thinner?" It's true that calories are important and that the only way to decrease actual body tissue weight is to take in fewer calories than are burned for energy. But though calories are important, they are not the only thing to consider when dieting.

Overall nutrition is of utmost importance for successful dieting. After all, dieting and your new slim stature should *improve* your health – not risk it.

To achieve and maintain good health, whether dieting or not, the human body requires certain proteins, fats and carbohydrates. Fluid, electrolytes and fiber are also essential – not to mention vitamins and minerals.

This chapter will briefly discuss these aspects of nutrition. It will be clear that *The World's Most Convenient Diet* is a safe plan that will help you reach a desired weight and add to your good health. It will also make you more informed about nutrition so you can better evaluate other diets you may have considered.

Protein

In order for any diet to be nutritionally sound, it must include adequate amounts of protein. But how much protein is adequate?

The National Academy of Science Food and Nutrition Board recommends a little less than one gram of protein for each two pounds of ideal body weight. However, it has been established that this estimate is roughly double the actual amount needed for a healthy person. The higher amount is given to assure adequate protein despite minor variances among individuals.

Why is protein important? Protein is necessary to maintain healthy body tissues, including muscles, skin and hair. It is also essential for hormone, enzyme and antibody formation. Many people think that exercise increases the need for protein, but this is not the case. Carbohydrates should be the source of energy needed for exercise.

Proteins are made up of amino acids, and it is the various amino acid combinations that build the body's different protein-containing tissues. The proteins that contain the best combination of amino acids for building tissue are called "complete proteins," and they come from animal foods. Beef, pork, fish, poultry and other meats, eggs, milk and milk products such as cheese and yogurt are the best sourcs of "complete" protein.

Protein is also found in dried beans and peas, as well as nuts. The quality of the protein is not quite as high as it is from animal foods, but these products can make an important contribution to a healthy protein intake when combined with certain grains and vegetables.

The World's Most Convenient Diet includes all these protein sources. Glance through the breakfast menus and you will notice milk, yogurt, eggs and foods containing eggs, such as waffles and French toast.

Lunches and dinners include beef, veal, ham, turkey, pork, chicken, cod, scallops, shrimp and additional seafoods, plus a wide variety of other sources of good protein. So anyone who has a doctor's approval to lose weight should not worry about the protein content of *The World's Most Convenient Diet*.

Fats

Many dieters assume fats are bad and should be avoided at all costs. It is true that fats are the most concentrated sources of calories and that a person will gain weight if he eats fats in an amount that exceeds his caloric needs. But the key word is the *amount* of fat. *The World's Most Convenient Diet* does limit fat, but does not eliminate it.

First of all, what are the sources of fat in food? Foods that are essentially 100 percent fat are butter, margarine and oils. Salad dressings, mayonnaise, cream, cream cheese, yogurt, milk, cheese, meats, gravy, nuts and peanut butter all contain significant amounts of their calories from fat.

You can lose weight on *The World's Most Convenient Diet* because the caloric intake from fats is controlled in the following ways:

1. Portion sizes of high-fat foods are limited. Low-calorie salad dressing is limited to one tablespoon per serving. Cream cheese, mayonnaise, gravy, peanut butter and all other fats are to be used only in specified amounts.
2. Whole milk is not permitted. Instead, low-fat milk, meaning milk that has two percent or less fat content, is required. Using skim milk is optional and would result in an even lower fat intake.
3. No cream is permitted for coffee or tea. If you need to have a dairy product added to your hot beverage, select a menu including low-fat milk and save some of the milk to add to your coffee or tea.
4. The amount of fat in each menu has not exceeded a predetermined level. By following the recommended portion size, approximately one-third of your day's calorie intake will come from fat.

Fats are important in the diet because they provide essential fatty acids that are necessary for healthy skin, nerves and cell structure. They also aid in absorbing fat-soluble vitamins and add flavor to food. This is why we do not believe fats should be eliminated or even *overly* restricted on a weight-reduction diet. They serve important nutritional functions and make the diet taste even better.

Nutrients

Carbohydrates

Carbohydrates are an important source of energy. Simple carbohydrates, such as sweets, provide "instant" energy because they are quickly absorbed and used by the body. Complex carbohydrates – starches – also provide energy, but over a longer time span.

Carbohydrates are essential for the optimal functioning of the central nervous system. Having enough calories from carbohydrates will also spare protein so that protein can be used for enzyme building, tissue repair and its other specific functions rather than being wasted on energy production.

If the body does not receive an adequate amount of carbohydrates, it can go into an unhealthy state known as "ketosis." This occurs when fats are metabolized too rapidly and accumulate in the blood in a form that is incompletely oxidized.

Some diets deliberately limit carbohydrates to create ketosis, resulting in a dangerously rapid weight loss. In extreme cases, ketosis can result in coma and even death. *The World's Most Convenient Diet* does not result in ketosis. It has been planned to assure adequate amounts of carbohydrates.

What are the sources of carbohydrates in *The World's Most Convenient Diet?* Grain products, fruits, vegetables and some sweets provide the nutrient.

If you select any one of the more than 300 menus on *The World's Most Convenient Diet*, you will find several sources of carbohydrates. For example, let's examine a sample breakfast from the "Ready to Eat Cereals" section:

¾ cup *Kellogg's® Special K®*
1 teaspoon sugar
½ cup low-fat milk
1 slice whole wheat, rye or white toast or
½ English muffin or
½ bagel
1 teaspoon margarine
1 choice from The Fresh Fruit Stand

The grain products in this meal are the cereal and the toast, English muffin or bagel. Carbohydrates from grain products are the starches, called complex carbohydrates. Other carbohydrate sources in the meal are the fruit, sugar and milk. Milk is also a source of fat and protein.

In summary, a good diet will include adequate carbohydrates because they are essential sources of energy and save protein so it can be used for more important jobs. Carbohydrate foods can also be important as sources of fiber. This will be discussed further in the section dealing with fiber.

Fluid And Electrolytes

The human body is approximately two-thirds water! Water is a key component in many body tissues and fluids. It rinses away waste products and regulates body temperature through evaporation. This should help you realize how important it is to have adequate amounts of fluids in your diet.

The World's Most Convenient Diet includes tap water, soda water, mineral water, sugar-free pop, coffee and tea as fluid sources.

Some unsafe weight-reduction diets limit fluids in order to create a false sense of weight loss. They may even encourage the use of diuretics ("water pills") that only add to the health risk. Consuming inadequate fluids certainly will result in weight decrease – but only temporarily. At best, the weight will return as soon as necessary fluids are consumed. At worst, the tactic could result in dangerous dehydration. Remember, permanent weight loss occurs only by the breakdown of solid tissues, not by mere loss of body fluids.

Sodium

Sodium is a mineral found naturally in food, table salt and some additives. Its purpose in the body includes regulating water balance and influencing nerve and muscle functions. Few people receive inadequate amounts of sodium in their diets. In fact, most people receive more sodium than necessary. For this reason, we do not recommend table salt be added to the foods in *The World's Most Convenient Diet*.

Potassium

Potassium is another important mineral involved in nerve and muscle function as well as acid-base and water balance. Potassium is widely available in foods, being found in milk, meats, poultry, seafood, whole grain breads and cereals and fruits and vegetables. A random check of any menu on *The World's Most Convenient Diet* will demonstrate many sources of potassium.

Chloride

Chloride is primarily obtained through table salt, which is chemically known as sodium chloride. As we mentioned, *The World's Most Convenient Diet* contains adequate amounts of salt, so no extra salt need be added.

Chloride has several functions. Primarily it is involved in acid-base balance and is a component of gastric juices needed for normal digestion of food.

Fiber

Fiber has received much attention recently as being an essential component of a healthy diet. There has been much talk about the connection between a high-fiber diet and the decreased risk of coronary heart disease, cancer of the colon, irritable bowel syndrome and diverticular disease. Increasing the diet's

Nutrients

fiber content generally will increase the number of bowel movements a person may have, but there is no conclusive evidence yet that this will make a person healthier.

A diet that contains a variety of foods, including fruits and vegetables, some whole grain bread or cereal products and adequate fluid, should result in "normal" bowel movements. It should be stressed that what is "normal" varies greatly among individuals.

The World's Most Convenient Diet offers a wide variety of foods, and this in itself should provide adequate fiber for most people. If, however, you would like to further increase fiber intake, you may select all your breads and cereals from those that are whole grains and eat extra allowed raw vegetables. Choosing prunes, raisins and dried apricots as some of your Fresh Fruit Stand selections may also help. In addition, these cereals on the diet are especially high in fiber:

Kellogg's® All-Bran®
Kellogg's® Bran Buds®
Kellogg's® Cracklin' Oat Bran™
Kellogg's® Fruitful Bran™
Nabisco® 100% Bran Cereal
Ralston® Bran Chex®
Any brand of raisin bran or 40% bran

Vitamins And Minerals

The World's Most Convenient Diet has been designed to provide maximum nutrition in combination with ease of preparation. We recommend a vitamin-with-minerals supplement be taken while following *The World's Most Convenient Diet* because, although most nutrients will be adequately supplied through the diet's wide variety of foods, the supplement will make up for any insufficiencies resulting from the decreased calorie level.

High doses of some vitamins and minerals can be toxic. For example, high doses of Vitamin D are known to cause kidney damage, while excess Vitamin A may harm the nervous system. Minerals taken in large amounts may result in complications not only due to their excess, but also because different minerals competing for the same absorption sites may not be as efficiently used. For these reasons, please select your vitamin-with-minerals supplement from our recommended list or use a generic equivalent.

Vitamins

For our discussion, vitamins will be divided into those that are fat-soluble and those that are water-soluble. The fat-soluble vitamins can be saved so the body can use them as the need arises. Water-soluble vitamins, however, cannot be efficiently stored. When amounts in excess of the current need are ingested, they are rinsed away in the urine. So it is important to receive adequate amounts of water-soluble vitamins in the diet each day.

Fat-Soluble Vitamins

Vitamin A

Vitamin A is important for maintaining healthy mucous membranes and skin, visual acuity in low light and the proper development of bones and teeth. Sources in the diet include fortified margarine, low-fat milk, cheese made from whole milk, egg yolks and vitamin enriched cereals.

Carotene, which the body can make into Vitamin A, is found in plants. Yellow or orange fruits and vegetables and dark green leafy vegetables are the best sources of carotene.

Vitamin D

Vitamin D is important for developing healthy bones and teeth by regulating the absorption of calcium and phosphorus. It is primarily supplied in the diet from milk, fortified cereals and margarine. Small amounts are found in egg yolks. An unusual quality of Vitamin D is that it can be synthesized in skin that has been exposed to ultraviolet light. So Vitamin D can be made in the body by sunlight.

Vitamin E

Vitamin E has been touted by some as increasing sexual prowess. While research has not substantiated this claim, Vitamin E is known to have a protective effect on red blood cells, Vitamin A, carotenes and polyunsaturated fatty acids. Animal foods (meats, poultry, fish, milk, etc.) are poor sources of this vitamin. Nuts, legumes, vegetable oils and green leafy vegetables are among the best sources of Vitamin E.

Vitamin K

The function of Vitamin K is to assure appropriate clotting time for blood by its involvement with the formation of prothrombin.

Good dietary sources are green leafy vegetables. Vitamin K can also be synthesized in the liver.

Water-Soluble Vitamins

Vitamin C

Vitamin C, known chemically as ascorbic acid, has many functions in the body. It aids in absorbing iron, keeps cartilage and capillary walls strong, helps prevent bleeding gums and excessive bruising and aids in developing

Nutrients

bones and teeth. A severe deficiency results in a disease known as scurvy. *The World's Most Convenient Diet* makes many sources of Vitamin C available. Among these are citrus fruits, strawberries, melons, potatoes, tomatoes, cabbage, green pepper and broccoli.

B-Complex Vitamins

B-Complex Vitamins received their name because of their interrelated functions and simultaneous appearance in foods. It is therefore unusual for a person to be deficient in only a single B vitamin. Thiamine (B^1), riboflavin (B^2) and niacin have roles in energy metabolism, cell respiration, the nervous system and enzymes.

Another B vitamin is B^{12} (cobalamin). Its functions include involvement with forming red blood cells, DNA and RNA.

While the B vitamins can be found in meats, vegetables and grain products, B^{12} generally occurs only in animal foods. So total vegetarians (people who don't eat meat, fish, eggs or milk products) may need to take a Vitamin B^{12} supplement.

Folic Acid

Like B^{12}, folic acid (or folate) is another important vitamin involved in preventing anemia by helping red blood cells mature properly. Folic acid also acts as a coenzyme and assists in forming all proteins. It can be found in meats, eggs, whole grain cereals and dark green leafy vegetables.

Minerals

Calcium

Most people know that calcium is needed for healthy bones and teeth. But calcium has many other functions in the body. Calcium is important for muscles, including the heart, to work properly. It also activates enzymes and helps transmit nerve impulses.

Milk, cheese, yogurt, cottage cheese, salmon (with bones) and some dark green leafy vegetables (turnip, collard and mustard greens, kale and broccoli) are among the best sources of calcium.

Phosphorous

Phosphorous works with calcium to create the structure of teeth and bones and it also has some less well-known functions. Phosphorous is found in the structural link of DNA and RNA. It is involved with carbohydrate and fat energy metabolism, the transport of fats as phospholipids and in the body's acid-base balance. Phosphorous is found along with calcium in most milk products and also in meats, eggs, whole grain products, nuts and legumes.

Magnesium

While we are discussing minerals essential to bone and tooth development, we must not overlook magnesium. As does calcium, magnesium influences nerve and muscle irritability and is also involved with carbohydrate metabolism. Cereals, nuts, legumes, meat and milk are the significant dietary sources of this mineral.

Iron

Iron is well known as an important mineral for preventing anemia. This is because it is an essential element in hemoglobin, which is found in red blood cells. Iron also functions as a component of several oxidative enzymes.

It is often difficult for women to obtain a sufficient quantity of iron from food. This is true even for women who are not on a weight-reduction diet. Because iron is lost during the menstrual cycle, a supplement is generally recommended for women of child-bearing age.

Dietary sources of iron include liver, meats, egg yolk, enriched and whole grain cereals and breads, legumes and dark green vegetables. Iron is best absorbed when taken in combination with foods containing vitamin C.

Zinc

This is another nutrient important to enzyme systems. In addition, it is involved with cell growth and wound healing. Fish and meat are good dietary sources of zinc. Plant foods, except for wheat germ and yeast, are generally low in zinc.

Chapter Nine
Supermarket Savvy

121	The Produce Department
133	Stocking the Cupboard
134	The Refrigerator and Freezer Sections

Supermarket Savvy

Today's grocery stores certainly are different from those even in the recent past. The tremendous variety of items continues to grow – especially among the convenience foods! Today as never before, both men and women are demanding easy-to-prepare foods to go along with their modern lifestyles. They don't want to spend extra hours in the kitchen when they could be playing racquetball, visiting their friends and families or just reading a book.

Convenience foods are looking and tasting better all the time. They have become so popular that grocers are having trouble keeping their shelves stocked. And convenience foods are now available in such a variety that menu possibilities are endless. This tremendous variety, however, can be a mixed blessing. It's wonderful to have so many choices, but how do you know where to start?

This chapter will help you enjoy your trip to the supermarket by making you more knowledgeable about your selections. After returning home, you will also be familiar with various storage techniques to help maintain the quality of what you've purchased.

First, we'll take you to the produce department, then on to select canned foods and other shelf items. Finally, we'll visit the refrigerator and freezer sections. After that, all that's left is the trip home to enjoy some delicious eating!

The Produce Department

Does broccoli scare you? Do you choose your cantaloupe with false assurance while secretly praying that it will be truly edible? When buying already prepared foods, you can count on the brand-name manufacturers to provide a quality product, but you're on your own when selecting fresh produce. Now fear no more. Not only will *The World's Most Convenient Diet* take you from "thick to thin," it will also bring you a new air of confidence in the produce department! Read on and become such a fruit and vegetable expert that your friends will be *plum* envious.

First let's examine some fruit . . .

Apples Apples of one type or another are available all year, but the time to buy the highest quality apples is in the fall. Purchase apples that are firm and have a good color. These apples generally will have improved flavor and keep longer. Apples that are soft will have a mealy texture when eaten and may spoil quickly.

Apples can be stored a variety of ways. First, however, separate those with bruises or skin breaks from the remaining apples.

Apples that are very ripe may be a bargain, but they need to be stored in the refrigerator and eaten within a week. Apples may be stored, although for not as long, at a room temperature of 60 to 70 degrees.

Apricots The time to purchase the best fresh apricots is in June or July. Look for fine golden-orange apricots that will yield to gentle pressure on the skin. Greenish or yellow apricots are not at the appropriate stage of ripeness and may not have good flavor. Apricots may be stored in the refrigerator for up to three to five days.

Bananas Bananas are available all year. The banana is one fruit whose flavor develops best if it is picked while not yet ripe. The green bananas should then be kept at room temperature (60 to 70 degrees) until they develop a yellow color with brown speckles. Do not buy bananas with bruises or dull grayish peels. Once ripe, bananas can be stored in the refrigerator. Although the skin will turn brown, the fruit inside remains good.

Blackberries, Boysenberries and Raspberries These berries are generally available during the summer months. No matter what type you select, make sure they are plump and firm. They should not be leaking, so check the container for signs of juice stains. The berries should be stored unwashed and uncovered in the refrigerator. Use within one to two days.

Blueberries The peak season for blueberries is June through August. The berries should be a very dark blue. Lighter colored berries will not be as flavorful. Select those that are plump and firm. Refrigerate then unwashed and uncovered. Eat them within two or three days because they, too, perish quickly.

Strawberries The prime season for strawberries is April through June. Look for medium-sized berries that are bright red with the caps and stems still attached. Larger berries may look attractive, but they are generally not as flavorful. Avoid berries that are soft and leaky and have large pale or green areas. Refrigerate the berries and eat them within one or two days.

Cantaloupe Melons The prime time for purchasing cantaloupes is late summer, but they may be available in stores from May until December. When selecting a cantaloupe, check for several signs:

1. Smell the cantaloupe. It should have a pleasant odor.
2. Check the shallow spot at the end of the melon where the stem has been. No fragment of skin should be remaining.
3. Look at its skin color. It should be a pale yellowish shade, not green (unripe) or dark yellow (overripe).
4. Feel the netting that covers the surface. It should be thick and stand out from the pale yellow background.
  Melons can be left at room temperature for a few days of complete ripening. They can be chilled prior to eating, if desired.

Cherries Sweet and sour cherries are in season during the summer

Supermarket Savvy

months. Most sour varieties are processed for pies and other desserts and are seldom sold on the retail market.

Look for plump, shiny cherries with a dark, rich color. Avoid those with either a dried or leaky, overripe appearance. Store them unwashed in the refrigerator for three days to two weeks.

Cranberries The peak season for cranberries is October through December. Choose firm, bright red berries. Sort out any leaky or damaged ones before eating. Cranberries are generally very sour and will require an artificial sweetener. Store them unwashed, but covered in the refrigerator for one to two weeks.

Dates Fresh dates are rarely available except from August until February in California. Look for dark brown, plump dates with smooth skin. Packaged dates can be stored unopened at room temperature for several months. Once opened, they can be covered again and refrigerated for one to two months.

Grapefruit Although actually in season from October through April, high-quality grapefruit can be purchased year round. A good grapefruit should feel heavy for its size. Grapefruits with thin skin are juicier than those with thick or rough skin. Avoid grapefruits with discoloring, wrinkles or other skin defects. Grapefruits can be stored at cool temperatures for at least two weeks.

Grapes The peak season for grapes is July through October. Grapes are of the red, white or green variety. Look for red grapes that are primarily red and white or green grapes that actually have a yellowish cast. The stems should be green and firmly attached to the grapes. The grapes should be plump, but not leaking.

Honeydew melon The best honeydew melons are available in June through September. A honeydew can be quite large (up to eight pounds), with a smooth, creamy-white rind. Do not buy a honeydew with dull white or greenish-white color because it is immature and will not sweeten. Also, avoid melons with injured rinds or soft, watery areas. A ripe melon can be refrigerated up to one week.

Mangoes Mangoes may be purchased from June until September. Look for those with a yellow-orange to red skin that yields slightly to pressure.

Nectarines Look for nectarines during July and August. The surface can have red shading or be completely red. A good nectarine should be plump and bright. Allow it to soften slightly at room temperature if it is purchased while still hard. Avoid shriveled or dull-colored nectarines.

Oranges Your best buys in oranges will occur during the fall and winter. Select oranges that are heavy and firm. The skin should be somewhat smooth, but skin color is not necessarily an indicator of high quality. Weakened areas of the skin or a dull, dry appearance are undesirable. Oranges may be refrigerated or stored at room temperature.

Papayas The peak season for papayas is from May until June. A good papaya will have a yellow-to-orange color and a skin that yields to gentle pressure. A green papaya can ripen at room temperature, but should not be placed in the sun. A ripe papaya can be stored uncovered in the refrigerator for up to three days.

Peaches Fresh peaches may be available from May to October. A good peach should be slightly soft but show no tan spots or bruises. The color should be bright, with a yellow or creamy appearance. A hard, green peach can be ripened at room temperature if kept away from sunlight. Riper peaches can be refrigerated unwashed for one to two weeks.

Pears Because there are several varieties of pears, one type or another is generally available from August through May. All types should be firm and free from dull, spotted skin and wilting. Check for these skin colors in the following varieties:
Anjou or Comice: yellow-green
Bartletts: pale to dark yellow
Boscs: green-yellow to brown yellow
Nelis: light to medium green
Pears can be ripened at room temperature, but should then be refrigerated.

Pineapples The prime season for pineapples is March through May, although they are marketed year round in most areas. Good pineapples will have a pleasant odor, be golden-yellow or reddish brown, depending on the variety, and have leaves that pull out easily. They should be plump and heavy without any trace of mold or shrinkage.

If not yet ripe, they should be left at room temperature. Otherwise, they may be wrapped and refrigerated for one to two days.

Plums Fresh plums are available in late May and mid-September. Plums should be slightly soft but without breaks in the skin or shriveling. The color will vary from green to reddish purple, depending on the variety. Avoid plums with breaks in the skin or bruising. Plums can be ripened at room temperature and then covered and refrigerated. Once ripe, they should be used as soon as possible.

Tangerines Tangerines are available from late November until early March. Select those with a yellow-orange color and intact skin. Because the skin is loose fitting, the tangerine may not feel firm but may still be good. However, avoid those with pale or punctured skin or soft spots. Store them in a cool place and use as soon as possible.

Watermelon The best time to buy watermelon is during the summer months. It is sometimes difficult to determine a high-quality melon by its outward appearance, but look for one with rounded ends and a creamy color on the "belly." A cut melon should have firm, red flesh with black or dark brown seed.

Supermarket Savvy

It should be juicy and free from white streaks and white seeds. An uncut watermelon may be refrigerated for at least one week. Once cut, it should be covered and stored for only one to two days.

And now for the vegetables . . .

Alfalfa sprouts Alfalfa sprouts should be fresh and springy. The leaves will be a light green and the stems will be a cream color. They should not be limp or showing signs of decay.

Asparagus Asparagus is available beginning in mid-February and ending in June. Look for asparagus that has smooth, brittle, deep green spears. The tips should be closed, with no sign of mold or vertical ridges. Check for excessive amounts of sand that could make washing difficult. Store it unwashed in the refrigerator for up to four days. Break off the tough lower end before eating.

Bean sprouts Bean sprouts should be a light creamy color and appear crisp. They should not show brown spots or decay or look wilted.

Beans, green or wax The peak season for green or wax "snap" beans is May through October. Choose slender beans that are crisp and bright colored. The length of the beans is not important, but avoid those with large seeds because they may have an undesirable mealy texture. Green or wax beans may be covered and refrigerated, washed or unwashed, for three to five days.

Broccoli Broccoli is available most of the year, except during the late summer months. Select broccoli that is deep green. Good broccoli can even be so dark that it appears purple. The clusters of buds should be tightly closed, showing no yellow flowers. Broccoli should be firm, but with stems that are not too thick or tough. It can be covered and stored in the refrigerator for three to four days.

Brussels sprouts The peak season for brussels sprouts is October through December, although they can be purchased during most of the year. Good brussels sprouts have bright green, tight-fitting outer leaves. Avoid those that have a yellowish color or holes in the leaves.

Cabbage Good cabbage is available all year. Choose cabbage with either a healthy looking red or green color, depending on the variety of cabbage. The head should be firm and heavy, without numerous blemishes or separation of the stem at the base. Most cabbage in the store has been trimmed of its outer leaves. If the leaves are present, however, check that they are not wilted, yellow or showing signs of worm injury. A fresh uncut head of cabbage can be refrigerated for several days.

Cabbage, Chinese Chinese cabbage is available all year. Select those with light green leaves that are crisp and free from any sign of decay.

Carrots Carrots are available throughout the year. Select those that are smooth, with a rich orange color. The carrots should be firm and free from wilting, cracks or spots of decay. Thin carrots may be sweeter than thick carrots. Carrots may be stored in the refrigerator for several weeks.

Cauliflower Cauliflower is available all year, but the peak season is September through January. Choose cauliflower that is compact and does not have spreading flowerets. The color should be white or a creamy white shade. Leaves growing through the flowerets do not affect the taste. Cauliflower may be refrigerated for up to five days if kept in plastic or in a crisper.

Celery Celery is available year round. Choose celery with thick, crisp stalks. Avoid celery that is cracked, limp or has brown discolorations. Freshness can be restored slightly if the bottom end is placed in water.

Chives Look for grasslike blades with a fresh green color. Avoid wilted, yellowed chives. Store them in a cold, humid section of your refrigerator.

Cucumber Cucumbers are available all year, but have a peak season from May to August. Select cucumbers that are firm, with an even shape and good green color. Cucumbers that are too large, yellow, puffy or shriveled may not taste good. Cucumbers may be stored in the refrigerator one to two weeks.

Endive (Chicory) and Escarole These greens can generally be purchased all year. Look for those that are fresh looking, with a bright green color and crisp leaves. Do not buy greens with blemishes, wilted leaves or coarse stems.

Kohlrabi The peak seasons for this member of the cabbage family are summer and fall. Purple and white (actually light green) kohlrabies are grown in this country, but the white is more popular. Both the fleshy stem and bulbar enlargement at the root end are edible. Kohlrabi is used chiefly as a cooked vegetable, but it can be eaten raw. You may be tempted to buy large kohlrabies, but the best ones are young and therefore not over three inches is diameter. Store kohlrabi at room temperature or in the refrigerator.

Lettuce Lettuce is available in several varieties, and one type or another can be purchased throughout the year. All varieties should be thoroughly washed and drained, then refrigerated in a plastic bag or crisper. When preparing your salad, tear rather than cut the leaves to prevent the edges from darkening.

Butterhead (includes Bibb and Boston lettuce) Look for small, loose lettuce heads with a rosette or cup shape. The leaves should be smooth and tender with a light green color.

Iceberg This lettuce should be in a round, solid head with crisp leaves. The outer leaves will be a darker green than the pale inner leaves. There should be no ragged brown areas.

Leaf There are several types of leaf lettuce and the color may vary from reddish to dark or pale green, depending on the variety. The leaves should be broad and tender.

Supermarket Savvy

Romaine or Cos Several different varieties of this lettuce are available. The leaves should be crisp and dark green. They are loosely folded in a cylindrically shaped head.

Mushrooms Mushrooms are available all year, with a slight decline in August. There are many types of mushrooms, but only one major type is marketed commercially. Fresh mushrooms should be white to very light brown in color. The caps should be closed so that few gills are exposed. The gills should be a light tan. Avoid mushrooms that are discolored or have a spongy texture. Do not soak mushrooms because they will rapidly absorb water. Instead, clean them quickly under running water. There is no need to peel them.

Onions There are many types of onions and some types are available all year. In general, select onions that are hard, with dry, papery skins. The necks should be small, with no sign of sprouting.

Scallions (green onions) Scallions are very young green onions that are available from May to August. They should have a fresh green color free from yellowed, wilted tops. Keep them in the refrigerator humidor and use them as soon as possible.

Parsley Parsley availability peaks in October through December, but it is generally available all year. Buy crisp, bright leaves that may be curled or flat, depending on the variety. Avoid parsley that is yellow, brown or wilted. Wash parsley in cold running water and refrigerate in the humidor.

Sweet Peppers Peppers are available all year, with a peak in June through September. Buy heavy, firm, brightly colored peppers. They may be green or red, but shape is not important. Avoid wilted peppers with cracks or soft spots. After washing and drying, they may be refrigerated in a plastic bag or crisper for three to five days.

Radishes The season for radishes peaks in May through July, but they are available all year. The most common radish is the round red variety, but there are also round white radishes and elongated white or red ones. Select medium-sized radishes that are firm and smooth, free from black spots or decay. Radishes that are overly large may have a spongy texture. Also, avoid radishes with yellowed tops. Radishes may be refrigerated for several days.

Spinach Spinach is available all year. Select spinach with a fresh green color free from wilting, decay spots and coarse stems. To store spinach, rinse well in cold running water. Then drain and refrigerate it in a covered container for as long as three to five days.

Squash, summer Some types of summer squash are available all year, not just during the summer months. Varieties include green zucchini, yellow crookneck and yellow straightneck. Look for summer squash that is glossy and firm, but not hard. Overmature squash will have a dull appearance. Squash does not need to be peeled to be eaten and can be used for salads as you would a cucumber. Keep it refrigerated and eat it as soon as possible.

Tomatoes Tomatoes are available all year, but good vine-ripened tomatoes can only be purchased in July through September in most parts of the country. Buy plump, firm tomatoes with rich color. Avoid those that are soft or cracked. Tomatoes can be ripened at room temperature and then refrigerated for a few days. Actually, tomatoes are a fruit, but most people think of them as a vegetable.

Watercress Watercress is available most of the year. Select watercress that has crisp, green leaves free from yellow or wilting. Watercress may be washed with cold water and stored for a day or two in the refrigerator.

Seasonal Availability of Produce

This chart can be used as a quick reference for selecting fresh fruits and vegetables. The produce is listed according to typical seasonal availability, which usually indicates when the highest quality foods can be obtained at the lowest prices. Keep in mind, though, that seasonal availability can vary from year to year depending on weather conditions.

Supermarket Savvy

Produce Seasonal Availability Chart

	January	February	March
Fruit	Apples*	Apples*	Apples*
	Bananas	Bananas	Bananas
	Grapefruit*	Grapefruit*	Grapefruit*
	Oranges	Oranges	Oranges
	Pears	Pears	Pears
	Tangerines	Tangerines	Pineapples
			Tangerines
Vegetables	Broccoli	Asparagus	Asparagus
	Cabbage	Broccoli	Broccoli
	Chinese cabbage	Cabbage	Cabbage
	Carrots	Chinese cabbage	Chinese cabbage
	Cauliflower	Carrots	Carrots
	Celery	Celery	Celery
	Lettuce and other greens	Lettuce and other greens	Lettuce and other greens
	Mushrooms	Mushrooms	Mushrooms
	Onions	Onions	Onions

continued

The World's Most Convenient Diet

	April	**May**	**June**
Fruit	Apples*	Apples*	Apples*
	Bananas	Bananas	Apricots
	Grapefruit*	Grapefruit*	Bananas
	Pears	Papaya	Blackberries
	Pineapple	Peaches	Blueberries
	Strawberries	Pears	Boysenberries
		Pineapples	Cherries
		Plums	Grapefruit*
		Strawberries	Honeydew melon
			Mangoes
			Papaya
			Peaches
			Plums
			Raspberries
			Strawberries
			Watermelon
Vegetables	Asparagus	Asparagus	Asparagus
	Broccoli	Beans, green	Beans, green
	Cabbage	or wax	or wax
	Chinese cabbage	Broccoli	Broccoli
	Carrots	Cabbage	Cabbage
	Celery	Chinese cabbage	Chinese cabbage
	Lettuce and	Carrots	Carrots
	other greens	Celery	Celery
	Mushrooms	Cucumber	Cucumbers
	Onions	Lettuce and	Kohlrabies
		other greens	Lettuce and
		Mushrooms	other greens
		Onions	Mushrooms
		Radishes	Onions
			Peppers
			Radishes

Supermarket Savvy

	July	**August**	**September**
Fruit	Apples*	Apples*	Apples*
	Apricots	Bananas	Bananas
	Bananas	Blackberries	Cantaloupe
	Blackberries	Boysenberries	Grapefruit*
	Blueberries	Cantaloupe	Grapes
	Boysenberries	Cherries	Honeydew melon
	Cantaloupe	Grapefruit*	Mangoes
	Cherries	Grapes	Peaches
	Grapefruit*	Honeydew melon	Pears
	Grapes	Mangoes	Plums
	Honeydew melon	Nectarines	
	Mangoes	Peaches	
	Nectarines	Pears	
	Peaches	Plums	
	Plums	Raspberries	
	Raspberries	Watermelon	
	Watermelon		
Vegetables	Beans, green or wax	Beans, green or wax	Beans, green or wax
	Cabbage	Cabbage	Cabbage
	Chinese cabbage	Chinese cabbage	Chinese cabbage
	Carrots	Carrots	Carrots
	Celery	Celery	Cauliflower
	Cucumbers	Cucumbers	Celery
	Kohlrabies	Kohlrabies	Kohlrabies
	Lettuce and other greens	Lettuce and other greens	Lettuce and other greens
	Mushrooms	Onions	Mushrooms
	Onions	Peppers	Onions
	Peppers	Radishes	Peppers
	Radishes	Squash	Squash
	Squash	Tomatoes	Tomatoes
	Tomatoes		

The World's Most Convenient Diet

	October	November	December
Fruit	Apples*	Apples*	Apples*
	Bananas	Bananas	Bananas
	Cranberries	Cranberries	Cranberries
	Grapefruit*	Grapefruit*	Grapefruit*
	Grapes	Oranges	Oranges
	Oranges	Pears	Pears
	Peaches	Tangerines	Tangerines
	Pears		
Vegetables	Beans, green or wax	Broccoli	Broccoli
	Broccoli	Brussels sprouts	Brussels sprouts
	Brussels sprouts		
	Cabbage	Cabbage	Cabbage
	Chinese cabbage	Chinese cabbage	Chinese cabbage
	Carrots	Carrots	Carrots
	Cauliflower	Cauliflower	Cauliflower
	Celery	Celery	Celery
	Kohlrabies	Kohlrabies	Kohlrabies
	Lettuce and other greens	Lettuce and other greens	Lettuce and other greens
	Mushrooms	Mushrooms	Mushrooms
	Onions	Onions	Onions
	Parsley	Parsley	Parsley

* Although apples and grapefruit are generally available all year, the highest-quality apples are found in the fall and grapefruits from October through April.

Supermarket Savvy

Stocking The Cupboard

Well, you've made it through the produce department so the hard part is over. Now you can sit back a little and rely on brand names to guarantee quality. But still, there are some general tips you need to know when stocking your cupboard.

Buy packages that look fresh. Labels that are torn or cans with dust could be a sign that the items are old. Inspect cans with dents to make sure no opening has been created and, of course, never buy a bulging can!

After the food has reached your home, store it in the coolest cupboards. Heat and humidity shorten shelf life. Many items have an expiration date printed on the container, so be sure to check it before eating the contents.

Please keep in mind that the maximum storage time for food being recommended here is to ensure good flavor and safety. By no means are we suggesting you should throw away foods that you may have had on your shelves longer than the ideal period. On the contrary, many canned foods are actually safe to use for years. In fact, food that has been recovered from family basements after sitting for more than 40 years has been found safe and nutritious! There are even reports of food recovered on the *USS Monitor* and the steamboat *Bertrand* that was still edible. By the way, both vessels sank in the 1860's!

Cereals If the package has not been opened, check the expiration date. Once opened, if the package liner is tightly closed after pouring, ready-to-eat cereal should stay fresh for up to three months.

Coffee Coffee's high price has made its purchase seem like a small investment! For this reason, it is wise to know what you are buying and how to store it.

There are many varieties of coffee, but don't assume that high price guarantees the best coffee. Buy what *you* like best. When purchasing ground coffee, select the grind that is suggested for your particular coffee maker. However, some brands of coffee do have a single grind that is recommended for drip, perk and electric coffee pots. Unopened vacuum-packed cans will keep the contents fresh for up to two years. Once opened, however, coffee should be refrigerated in a tightly closed container and used as soon as possible.

The shelf life of instant coffee is similar to that of vacuum-packed ground – up to two years if the container is unopened and a much shorter period once opened. This does not mean that the ground and instant coffee will be unsafe to drink after the recommended times have lapsed, but they will not have optimal flavor.

Mayonnaise An opened jar of mayonnaise can be stored for several months. Check the expiration date to be sure. Once opened, it must be refrigerated.

Salad Dressings Bottled salad dressing that has not been opened will keep for up to 12 months. Once again, check the expiration date to be certain.

Opened salad dressing can be refrigerated for up to three months. Dressings made from mixes generally should not be kept longer than a couple of weeks.

Syrups One year is the approximate shelf life of an unopened or opened bottle of syrup. Refrigerated, it will last even longer.

Tea Instant tea that is kept in a tightly covered container will last up to three years. Loose tea, also tightly covered, will keep its flavor for up to two years. Tea that is in bags has the shortest life, but it is still quite long – about 18 months.

Soup and Soup Mixes If kept in a cool and dry location, soups and soup mixes should last at least one year. Prepared soup should be refrigerated and eaten within a few days.

Canned Fruit Juices Keep canned fruit juice in a cool place and the contents should stay fresh for 8 to 10 months. Once opened, it should be refrigerated and used within one week.

Meat, fish and other seafood Unopened cans will keep one year. After opening, use the contents within two days. Incidentally, tuna is available in several varieties. If the tuna will be broken up to be mixed with mayonnaise or salad dressing, the flaked or grated style will save you time and money over the solid or chunk varieties.

Fruit Canned fruit, unopened, should be used within one year. Any leftover fruit can be refrigerated up to a week. Dried fruit can be kept fresh in an airtight container for six months. Refrigerating will ensure higher quality.

Catsup Unopened catsup will keep one year. After opening, it can be stored at room temperature for one month. It will last much longer if refrigerated.

Mustard Prepared yellow mustard can be stored unopened for two years and opened for several months. As with catsup, it may be refrigerated.

Peanut Butter Peanut butter may be stored for several months if unopened. After opening the jar, the flavor is best if it is used within a few months. Refrigerating helps with preservation, but makes the peanut butter difficult to spread! Remember to bring it to room temperature before using.

The Refrigerator And Freezer

We're almost finished and it's becoming easier, isn't it? We're approaching more items, this time from the refrigerator and freezer sections. Here are some tips for selecting and storing even more foods.

Supermarket Savvy

How well do you know your refrigerator? Did you know that the most important thing about your refrigerator is that its temperature should be kept between 34 and 40 degrees? If the temperature is too cool, foods can be ruined by freezing, and if the temperature is not cool enough, the growth of bacteria and molds can rapidly set in. If some food does start to spoil, it should be immediately removed or the spoiling can spread to other foods. In addition to the proper temperature, airtight containers or wraps are important to preserve food quality and wholesomeness.

The temperature of a freezer should be no higher than zero degrees. When in the grocery store, be sure to choose frozen foods just prior to leaving. The contents of the packages should be solidly frozen, with no frost collected on the outside. Frost could be an indication that the food has thawed and been refrozen. Place foods in your freezer as soon as you arrive home.

Keep in mind that the recommended storage lengths, as with the canned foods, don't mean you should throw out foods that have been in your freezer or refrigerator beyond the suggested dates. These are merely general recommendations for optimal freshness and flavor.

Margarine Margarine should keep well for at least five months at refrigerator temperatures, or it can be frozen for up to one year if kept moisture-free. Please note that this does not apply to whipped margarine, which should not be frozen.

Cheeses Cottage cheese will keep in the refrigerator for at least several days. It should not be frozen, however, because its texture will become mushy. Harder cheeses, such as brick, cheddar and Swiss, can be refrigerated unopened for up to six months. Once opened, they can be stored for three to four weeks if in a block, but only about two weeks if sliced. Always keep cheese tightly covered so that it will not become dry. Any surface mold can simply be cut away; it will not affect the flavor of the cheese or render it unsafe to eat. The harder cheeses can be frozen, though the color and texture may change slightly. This is not a problem if the cheese will be used for cooking, but if you plan to serve the cheese sliced or cubed at room temperature, it may crumble and appear less attractive than fresh cheese. Processed cheeses will keep for at least one month after opening. Some types do not even need to be refrigerated. As with all cheeses, always remember to keep them covered to prevent drying. Processed cheeses can also be frozen for up to three to four months.

Milk Fresh milk can be kept at least several days in the refrigerator if it's not allowed to reach room temperature during meals. For maximum storage life, pour your milk and immediately return the remainder to the refrigerator. Keep the container tightly closed and never pour unused milk back into the container. Milk can be frozen if it is used within one month. The color and flavor will be affected, so the thawed milk should only be used for baking and other cooking.

Eggs Fresh eggs can be kept at least three weeks in the refrigerator.

Unless they are used quickly, store them in their carton or another covered container rather than on the egg keeper found in many refrigerators. Eggshells are quite porous, so unless the eggs are covered they can actually lose moisture through the shells. If you want the yolks to be nicely centered when cooked, store them with the small end of the shell pointing downward. Whole eggs should not be frozen.

Yogurt Yogurt can be refrigerated for at least several days. Most cartons have an expiration date printed on them, so be sure to check it before purchasing the yogurt. Yogurt can be frozen, although it is not generally recommended.

Cured and Smoked Meats If your refrigerator has a section for storing meats, use it for all cured and smoked meat products. They should be kept tightly wrapped. If your refrigerator does not have such a specially designated area, store these meats in what appears to be the coldest part of your refrigerator.

Frankfurters, once opened, will keep at least one week. Luncheon meats will stay fresh at least three days. Freezing of cured or smoked meats is not recommended. They may become rancid or "weep" liquid. If they must be frozen, use them within one month.

Breaded Fish Breaded fish may be stored in a home freezer for at least three months. If only part of a package is used, be sure that the remaining portions are tightly sealed before they are returned to the freezer.

Fruit Juice Fruit juice concentrates in their original containers will maintain their quality for up to one year. Frozen fruit that is either purchased already frozen or is home frozen in moisture-proof containers can also be kept frozen for twelve months.

Vegetables Home frozen vegetables or those that are purchased already frozen will maintain their quality for eight to ten months. Not all vegetables will keep their fresh texture once they are thawed, so it is best to cook them from the frozen state.

Main Dishes Casseroles and frozen dinners are best if used within three months.

Baked goods Freezing will not make bakery products "fresher," but it can maintain the quality of the product at the time of freezing. Moisture-proof wrapping is especially important. If cooked properly, baked goods can be maintained for several months.

All done! Are you feeling better about your trips to the grocery store? Now picture yourself pushing the cart, with your new slim physique, while other shoppers are looking at you and your purchases. They'll glance at your pizzas, croissants and donuts while thinking, "Some people can eat whatever they want and still never have to worry about their weight!"

Chapter Ten
Diet Dialogue

Diet Dialogue

Anyone getting ready to embark on a diet should carefully examine the plan and fully understand how it works. We've anticipated some questions you might have about our diet's procedures, effectiveness, safety, cost and nutrition, and will answer them in our "diet dialogue."

How fast will I lose weight on your diet?
The speed of your weight loss will depend on several factors:
1. How much weight do you have to lose? If you are a good deal overweight, *The World's Most Convenient Diet* will yield a greater calorie reduction for you than someone who is smaller. Therefore, you will lose weight faster.
2. Have you increased your activity level? This will help burn calories and result in a more rapid weight loss.
3. Are you following the diet exactly? Extra food or between meal snacking will slow your progress.

Our clients who have followed *The World's Most Convenient Diet* have had losses of two to three pounds per week. It is not unusual for the first week weight loss to be three to five pounds. Look for a 9 to 11-pound weight loss each month.

How long do you recommend staying on your diet?
It's completely up to you! Stay on your diet until you reach the weight you want. Consult the recommended weight-for-height formula for guidance concerning an appropriate weight range. This appears in Chapter 7. (Note: Before starting any diet or exercise program, consult your physician.)

What special appliances will I need to follow the diet?
If you consider a refrigerator, range and perhaps a toaster standard equipment, then *no* special appliances are needed. Some menu items include package directions for preparing the food in a microwave, but this is by no means essential because alternate heating methods can be used. If lunch is eaten away from home and cooking facilities are not available, carry lunches in a thermos bottle if possible or select from the Fast Food Fare or Simple Sandwiches sections.

Do I need to buy a scale to follow your diet?
No! Simply check package weights for entrees to be sure they correspond, within one ounce, to the weight specified by the menu. Purchase cheese that's already sliced, if possible, and divide the package weight in ounces by the number of slices to determine weight per slice. Weights of other foods can be similarly calculated by comparing to the package weight and number of servings per package.

Is the diet expensive?
Only if you want it to be expensive – and even then you may find you are

spending less on groceries than you were before starting the diet. With more than 300 menus to select from, the amount you spend on entrees is really up to you. Here are some tips: To save money, select seasonal and less expensive items for the Super Salad Bar and Fresh Fruit Stand. Watch for specials on other menu items and use coupons for additional savings. Buy bread on sale and freeze it. For cereals where brand name is not specified, such as corn flakes and raisin bran, use generic varieties. Try generic peanut butter, too.

Does your program include the use of diet pills?
No! We believe they are unnecessary and do not help with *permanent* weight loss. Diet pills can also present a health risk in some instances. Our diet is a healthy, well-planned weight-reduction program that also teaches appropriate eating habits for weight-loss maintenance.

Will moderate alcohol intake affect my weight loss on this diet?
Yes – adversely. Although it is not necessarily unsafe for dieters, alcohol will slow down weight reduction or even prevent it altogether, depending upon your definition of "moderate." The reason is that with the exception of fat, alcohol is the most concentrated source of calories. Per gram, alcohol has a higher energy value than pure sugar! One ounce of liquor, such as bourbon, vodka, gin or rum, contains 80 to 100 calories. Add this to the calories of a mix and you have strayed significantly from your diet. Beer and wine are also sources of calories. Here are the average calorie contents of some popular alcoholic beverages:

Alcoholic Beverages	Calories
Highball-8 ounces	170
Manhattan-3½ ounces	165
Martini-3½ ounces	140
Old Fashioned-4 ounces	180
Tom Collins-10 ounces	180
Italian Vermouth-3½ ounces	170
Beer-12 ounces	150
Wine, Muscatel or Port-3½ ounces	160

The calorie content of alcoholic beverages is enough reason for avoiding them. In addition, however, there is the appetite stimulating effect of alcohol. A predinner cocktail can make what otherwise would be a satisfying meal seem insufficient – and may take away your will power to adhere to the meal plan.

I've tried counting calories in the past. I hated it! Do I have to do that on your diet?
No. All the counting has been done for you to make the diet as convenient as possible. We checked nutrient information from numerous food companies and then selected those items that could fit in our predetermined calorie limits. Those selected items then were placed in breakfast, lunch or supper menus. You

Diet Dialogue

simply choose three meals each day.

Will your diet prevent or cure disease?
Diabetes, heart and vascular diseases, hypertension, arthritis and varicose veins are among the health problems linked to obesity. While weight reduction cannot guarantee prevention or relief from these problems, it will almost always be beneficial.

How often should I weigh myself?
We recommend weighing only once each week. This is because your weight will fluctuate daily. Even during the same day, there will be differences because of recently ingested beverages or meals and changes in clothing. Choose a specific day and time each week and weigh yourself without clothing or with the same light clothing each time. Weighing first thing in the morning, before breakfast, might be the most encouraging. You may want to keep a graph of your weight loss on the refrigerator to admire in between weekly weigh-ins.

When I glanced at the menu selections, I noticed bread, potatoes, donuts, lasagna and pizza! How can I lose weight eating these foods?
Many people eat these foods and maintain a good weight. The secret is portion size. Be assured that as long as you follow the recommended portion size, your caloric intake should be low enough to cause a weight loss.

Are convenience foods nutritious?
Some convenience foods, such as soda pop and candy, contain only calories and are not nutritious in their vitamin, mineral and protein content. However, other convenience foods are very nutritious because they are made from meats, fish, vegetables, fruits, dairy products and enriched or whole grain flours. So properly *selected* and *combined* convenience foods certainly can make up a very nutritious meal plan. We've done all the investigative work for you so you can be sure that *The World's Most Convenient Diet* is nutritionally sound.

Aren't convenience foods high in calories but low in protein?
To answer your question, let's take a look at homemade beef stroganoff versus a frozen product. A homemade beef stroganoff dinner tallies up to 640 calories per serving, while one serving of *Green Giant®* Beef Strogonoff with noodles contributes 300 fewer calories!
After analyzing the nutrient data, you find you are actually getting fewer calories and more *protein per calorie* from the convenience product. An added bonus: Not only have you saved calories, you've saved time!

Occasionally I may not be able to follow the diet exactly due to being at a friend's home for dinner or when dining in a restaurant. What should I do?
We realize it may not be possible to follow the diet for every single

meal on every single day. When an exception to the diet is necessary, use these patterns: For lunch, substitute three ounces of broiled or baked lean meat, fish or poultry with fat or skin removed, one small roll or one slice whole wheat, rye or white bread with one teaspoon margarine, one trip to the Super Salad Bar and one choice from the Fresh Fruit Stand. For dinner, add one extra ounce of meat or fish.

Consult the Menu Planner section if specific meal suggestions are needed. This alternate meal plan can also be used when you are "in the mood" to cook.

Does this mean dining out is not taboo on this diet?
That's right. It's going to take some figuring out on your part, but if you follow the guide given in the previous question, you'll be okay. For example, it would be acceptable to order broiled sirloin with a roll and a salad and melon for dessert. Don't be afraid to ask how the food is prepared; in fact, be even more assertive – ask if it can be prepared *your* way.

What about holidays? There's almost always a small feast associated with them!
Holidays are always going to exist (thank goodness), so the sooner you learn to handle the feasting that accompanies them, the better you will be at reckoning with them. Don't let the holiday control you. Decide ahead of time what you will eat. Choose a breakfast from the menu planning section. Don't skip it because you'll be more likely to overeat later. For lunch and supper, you have the option of choosing a convenience meal or following the basic guideline for the nonconvenience meal. Do not make eating the main event of your holiday. Enjoy the company of family and friends and spend time getting acquainted or re-acquainted. A brisk walk at some time during the festivities often helps keep your mind off the food. Remember, the focus of the holiday should be enjoying others and all the activities, not eating.

I don't like eating breakfast or lunch, but in the evening – look out! Do I have to eat breakfast and lunch on your diet?
While the time of day that the three meals are eaten can be varied to suit your schedule, we *strongly* encourage the three meals be just that – three individual meals spaced throughout the day. Going for extremely long periods of time without eating generally results in a binge when you finally do eat. Your large food intake in the evening may be what causes you not to be hungry in the morning. Try eating three meals, plus some snacks from the allowed vegetables, and see if you feel better and are able to adhere to the diet.

Does exercise increase the need for protein?
No. Most people require less than one gram of protein for each two pounds of ideal body weight regardless of their exercise routine. A person exercising for reasons other than weight loss should receive extra calories from

Diet Dialogue

carbohydrates rather than protein.

Your diet includes pizza, hamburgers and tacos. Aren't those "junk foods?"

If by "junk foods" you mean foods devoid of protein, vitamins, minerals and other nutrients, the answer is a definite "No!" Let's examine these foods in terms of your basic food groups. They are:

1. Meat or meat substitute group
2. Fruit and vegetable group
3. Milk and milk products group
4. Bread and cereal group

First, consider pizza. Pizza crust is from the bread and cereal group; the cheese is from the milk group; tomato sauce and any vegetables, such as mushrooms, onions and green peppers, are from the fruit and vegetable group; and if the pizza has sausage and pepperoni, the meat group is also represented.

Now let's analyze hamburger. The hamburger patty is obviously from the meat group and the bun from the bread and cereal group. If cheese and lettuce and tomato are added, the milk and fruit and vegetable groups would also be included. The taco can also have ingredients from all four food groups. The taco shell is a grain product, so it is, of course, from the bread and cereal group. By now you can determine the foods groups represented by beef, cheese, lettuce and tomato.

In summary, pizza, hamburger, and tacos can be part of a well-balanced diet.

Is it best to get most of your calories from protein? I've heard about those "high-protein diets."

The primary function of protein is to provide amino acids (the "building blocks" of proteins) to build and repair the various protein-containing components of the body. When the majority of food intake comes from protein, it means that protein is being used for calories. This is a wasteful as well as expensive way to use protein! Carbohydrates and fats should be the primary source of calories in the diet. Diets promoting the exclusive intake of high-protein foods may even result in ketosis. This is the same unhealthy state of metabolism that can occur in people with uncontrolled diabetes. In addition, these high-protein diets may be very low in fiber and may not promote permanent healthy eating habits.

Won't including foods such as donuts, pasta, mashed potatoes and gravy teach dieters bad habits?

On the contrary, it teaches dieters how to include these popular foods in sensible amounts so that they may continue enjoying them long after they have reached their desired weight. We all know slim people who routinely eat those so-called forbidden foods. And how do they remain slim? It is because their total caloric intake does not exceed what their body needs. You see, there is really nothing intrinsically evil about donuts, pasta or even mashed potatoes and gravy.

Aren't convenience foods too salty?

Some convenience foods contain significant amounts of sodium (salt). We have prepared the menus for *The World's Most Convenient Diet* so that the daily sodium content will usually range from 2,000 to 3,500 milligrams if no additional salt or sodium-containing seasonings are added. Thirty-five hundred milligrams of sodium per day is actually considered a moderate sodium intake. The average American typically gets 6,000 to 10,000 milligrams of sodium daily.

I usually add salt to my foods. Can I continue doing this on your diet?

We do not recommend using additional salt. The convenience foods already contain a sufficient amount of sodium. Too much salt is a bad habit of many people and now would be a good time to stop. There are some good salt alternatives available today. We do not mean only salt substitutes; there are some excellent blends of herbs and spices that can now be purchased.

I noticed fast food items are included in the diet. Can I take a trip to the Salad Bar at these fast food places?

You certainly can. We ask that you familiarize yourself with the allowed raw vegetables in our own Super Salad Bar list and then limit your choices at the restaurant Salad Bar to those that are permitted. Remember, one tablespoon of diet dressing is allowed. If no diet dressing is offered, you might bring your own or use vinegar or lemon juice.

Why do you recommend I take a multivitamin-with-minerals pill?

We have designed *The World's Most Convenient Diet* to contain as many nutrients as possible. Meats, dairy products, fruits, vegetables and enriched grain and cereal products are *all* included. However, because it is a reduced-calorie diet, adding daily multivitamin-with-minerals pills will serve as added assurance that you are receiving essential nutrients.

What if I can't find the product listed in your menus?

If this should occur with one of your choices, don't be upset. There are more than 300 menus from which to choose. You could also ask your grocer to stock a particular item.

Don't manufacturers sometimes change the size of their product packages?

Companies do occasionally change a package size or an ingredient of a product. Try to buy package sizes that are within one ounce of the weight specified in the menu. If you are still in doubt, please choose an alternate meal from the extensive selections offered.

Diet Dialogue

I hate fish! Do I have to eat it on your diet?
Remember that *The World's Most Convenient Diet* has more than 300 menu selections. Our menus do include fish, but you certainly do not have to choose those particular menus if you do not prefer them. Even by eliminating the seafood entrees, you will still have plenty of variety.

I've been on a hundred different diets and have been unsuccessful because I've become bored with them all. If I never see another grapefruit or "diet milkshake," it will be too soon. Is your diet any different?
Definitely. You eat only the foods *you* like on *The World's Most Convenient Diet.* If you dislike grapefruit, then there is no reason for you to ever eat it! Our meal plans also do not depend on "diet milkshakes" or other liquid formulas. You select from the extensive list of breakfasts, lunches and dinners and eat only the foods you like.

I don't really need to lose weight, but I have to carefully watch what I eat to avoid gaining. Could I follow your diet for one or two days a week to help me maintain my current weight?
Certainly! That's the perfect solution to your weight maintenance program. If you happen to exceed your normal caloric allowance occasionally, following the diet for one or two days each week will help balance your total caloric intake to the appropriate amount.

I prefer not to eat pork for religious reasons. Would this present a problem on your diet?
Certainly not! Simply avoid the menus containing ham, bacon, sausage or any other pork products. Read the package ingredients if you have any question concerning the content of an entree. *The World's Most Convenient Diet* offers such a wide variety of menu selections that most specific food preferences can be accommodated.

Is this diet a good one for vegetarians?
If you are a true vegetarian who avoids all animal products, the diet will not offer enough menu selection for you. Some people who consider themselves vegetarians do eat seafood and occasionally even poultry. If this is the case with you, then *The World's Most Convenient Diet* certainly would be acceptable.

Can I follow your diet and still limit my intake of fat and cholesterol?
Yes. While *The World's Most Convenient Diet* is not meant to be therapeutic in that regard, only entrees meeting our criteria for controlled fat content were included. Fat is also limited through the use of low-fat or skim milk rather than whole milk or cream and by including only specific amounts of margarine, oils, salad dressings and other fats. In addition, you can increase the proportion of polyunsaturated to saturated fats in the diet by using margarines and oils made from safflower, sesame, sunflower or corn oils. Incorporating fewer saturated fats in products is a desirable trend in the food industry. Choles-

terol also can be limited by choosing egg breakfasts no more than two or three times per week, using margarine instead of butter and by selecting menus including fish and skinless poultry.

I've heard it's important to include fiber in my daily food intake. Can I do this on your diet?
Including adequate fiber in your diet is an excellent idea. We would recommend choosing bran cereals from the breakfast menus two or three times a week. Any bread you may need to use on this diet could be a whole grain type. Our Super Salad Bar list provides an array of fresh vegetables that will also add to the fiber content of your diet. Finally, the Fresh Fruit Stand offers a wide variety of fresh fruits that will add bulk. In addition to adding fiber to your diet, all of the suggestions are excellent vitamin sources.

May I use honey to sweeten my food?
Many people are under the impression that honey is low in calories. Actually, per tablespoon, honey has slightly more calories than regular sugar! Therefore, we do not recommend its use. Please use artificial sweeteners or the *specified amounts* of Aunt Jemima®Lite Syrup as sweetening agents.

Do you recommend fasting prior to starting your diet?
Fasting can be dangerous if it is not closely monitored by a physician. What's more, fasting is not necessary with our diet. On our program you can safely lose weight while still enjoying lasagna, chili, rolls, waffles and many other delicious treats. So why fast?

I think I'm overweight because of a thyroid problem. What should I do?
Check with your doctor. There are specific tests that can be done to determine if you truly do have an abnormal thyroid condition. But the percentage of people who are overweight because of this problem is extremely small. Most people are overweight because of a combination of under-activity and over-eating. Their attempts at weight loss fail because they make no significant changes in the practices that make them overweight in the first place. They may then blame their condition on a thyroid problem.

I know I eat less than many of my friends, but I'm overweight and they aren't. How can that be?
We need to ask you a couple of questions before we can answer. Do you really take in fewer calories than your friends? You may eat smaller meals, but what do they include? And what about between-meal snacks and beverages? Many people forget to consider these as sources of calories. If you are really taking in fewer calories, consider the amount of exercise you take. Studies have shown that often overweight people really do eat less, but they may spend less time participating in physical activities and more time sitting or sleeping than

Diet Dialogue

their slim counterparts. We suggest you faithfully adhere to our diet and increase your activity after first checking with your physician.

Your diet is fine, but so often I eat even when I am not hungry. Maybe it's nerves or boredom. What should I do?

Many people turn to food for reasons other than hunger. Relieving anxiety or boredom are just two reasons why many people may overeat. Identifying the underlying motivation for your eating and finding an alternate way of dealing with the problem will certainly help your dieting efforts.

Can you give me any tips to help me stay on the diet?

Here are a few suggestions to help you:

1. Plan your meals so that all needed items are available. This way you never have a reason to stray from the diet for even one meal.
2. Weigh yourself only one time each week – preferably the first thing in the morning before eating, drinking or getting dressed. This should be encouraging because you'll be checking yourself at your lightest weight. Weighing yourself more frequently is not a good idea because your weight may vary due to fluid intake and you may become discouraged.
3. Set realistic goals. We have said that on *The World's Most Convenient Diet* the average weight loss is three to five pounds the first week and two to three pounds in subsequent weeks. If you expect to lose weight much more rapidly, you will become discouraged. Remember, this diet results in a safe and steady weight loss and this is the type of weight most likely to *stay off*.
4. Get encouragement from family and friends. Studies have shown that dieters who receive support from others are more successful.

Finally, please consult the chapter "Taking You Through Thick to Thin" for more assistance in losing and keeping your weight off.

How can I identify a diet that may be nutritionally unsound?

Ask yourself these questions after studying the diet:

1. Does the diet emphasize only a few foods instead of encouraging a wide variety? A diet that limits your food selections will not ensure adequate nutrients. An extreme example of an unhealthy food plan is the macrobiotic diet that promotes the intake of brown rice exclusively in the diet's final stage.
2. Does the diet require the purchase of high-dosage vitamin/mineral supplements? A supplement containing the Recommended Daily Allowances (RDAs) or amounts close to them is a wise addition to a weight-reduction diet because caloric limitations may result in a slightly inadequate intake of some nutrients. However, a diet that promotes vitamins and minerals in amounts *far exceeding* the RDAs results in the dieter taking unnecessary supplements that are a waste of money and could even be potentially harmful.
3. Does the diet's promoter claim it *will cure* certain diseases? As we have

mentioned, there are certain health problems that can be helped or possibly prevented by maintaining an ideal body weight, a sound diet and exercise. However, any diet claiming to *absolutely* cure or prevent specific diseases cannot be accurate.
4. Does the diet make claims for rapid weight loss? A diet that states it will result in a rapid weight loss is either dangerously unsound or making false claims – or both! Extremely rapid weight loss is unhealthy and is generally the result of a "crash" diet or diet that severely limits fluids. These diets are unsafe unless prescribed by a physician to treat a specific medical condition.
5. Does the diet teach you how to eat after you have reached your desired weight? If not, you are sure to regain your lost weight! This is why so many people experience a "yo-yo-ing" weight. A good diet will include "normal" foods and teach you to be satisfied with appropriately sized portions.

These are only a few questions to ask yourself when trying to determine if a diet is sound. If you still have questions, consult a *registered* dietician.

I am the mother of three small children. I really want to work on shaping up my figure, and losing weight would certainly help. But how do I find the time to follow the diet?
Very little extra time is needed to follow our diet. Select your menus in advance so the necessary items can be obtained at the same time you buy food for the rest of your family. To make shopping even easier, think of foods that can be enjoyed by both you and other members of your family. Cereal, bread and items from the Fresh Fruit Stand and Super Salad Bar are a few examples. However, make sure the servings you require are *saved for you* and haven't already been eaten when you go to prepare your meals! The only items requiring special preparation are the entrees, and they are so easy to get ready that it is generally only a matter of slipping a container into the oven along with whatever is being prepared for the rest of your family. With three small children, you may not have the time to do many things – but you will be able to succeed following *The World's Most Convenient Diet*.

I am a bachelor who hates to shop and cook. Will your diet be as convenient for me?
This diet will be *perfect* for you and others who dislike shopping and cooking! Here's why:
1. The majority of foods on our diet are convenience items. This means you can limit your trips to the store by stocking up on enough menu selections to last for several weeks. Even bread can be kept in the freezer. If this is done, all additional shopping can be accomplished with a brief weekly trip to the store for milk and perhaps some items from the Fresh Fruit Stand or the Super Salad Bar. Remember, a shopping list for one week's worth of menus has already been prepared if you choose to use it. If not, you can use the same

Diet Dialogue

convenient format for writing your own shopping list.
2. Now that you realize how easy shopping can be, let's talk about cooking. It's even easier! All the menus in *The World's Most Convenient Diet* were specifically designed to make preparation as simple as possible. Most entrees have package sizes that result in *no leftovers*. Some, such as *Armour Dinner Classics®*, are packaged so that transferring the entree to a dinner plate is not even necessary. And, of course, entrees not packaged in a ready-to-eat style can always be served on disposable plates along with disposable utensils and cups! How much more convenient can you get? Well, we have one more suggestion. Do some advance preparation for the Super Salad Bar. Wash and prepare salad items ahead of time and refrigerate them in a plastic container with a tight-fitting lid. Salad preparation is then reduced to scooping a bowl full of salad! We do advise that you don't add dressing until you are ready to start eating.

I don't work a typical 9 to 5 schedule. My usual work day is midnight to 8 a.m. May I eat "supper" at 9:30 a.m.?
Certainly. As long as you adhere to our meal plans, they may be eaten at times most convenient for your daily routine. For example, it is perfectly acceptable for you to eat "breakfast" at 11 p.m. before work, "lunch" at 3 a.m. while at work and "supper" at 9:30 a.m. after work.

I'm six months pregnant and have gained a little too much weight so far. Can I follow your diet safely during my pregnancy to lose a few pounds?
Weight reduction during pregnancy is generally not advisable, even for someone who is quite a bit overweight. We suggest you follow the advice of your dietitian and doctor to control your weight gain for the remainder of your pregnancy. However, we do strongly recommend our diet to achieve weight loss *after* your delivery and any nursing period are over. Our diet can result not only in your reaching your pre-pregnancy weight, but an even lower weight, if you desire.

I'm a senior citizen who hates to cook meals for myself. Your diet looks great because the cooking is already done for me! But is your diet safe for me?
This diet can be an excellent choice for senior citizens. The ease of preparation, the single portions and the wide variety of meals are especially appealing. We ask that you check with your physician first. If you are not on a severe sodium restriction, this diet could be an excellent choice. A day's sodium total on *The World's Most Convenient Diet* would generally average 2,000 to 3,500 milligrams, a moderate level.

Is exercising all that important?
Yes! And here's why:
1. Exercise will burn calories to help you lose weight faster.
2. Exercise will help tone your muscles to give you the appearance of greater weight loss.
3. Exercise is a great substitute activity for eating. For example, taking a 20-minute walk instead of eating a piece of cherry pie will save you 500 calories – 400 from not eating the pie and 100 calories burned up walking! Enjoyed every day, this substitute activity in itself can result in an additional one pound weight loss each week!
4. Exercise is a great way to keep your spirits up. Try a congenial contest in tennis or racquetball and see if you don't feel better. There are many dance exercise programs for less competitive athletes. With the extra hour you now have before dinner (because preparation time is so short), join a neighborhood exercise spa. (Note: Always check with your doctor to learn what exercises are recommended for you.)

I'm working hard to lose weight. But in the meantime, how can I look thinner?
Changes in make-up, hairstyle and clothing can result in a thinner appearance. Try your local library for books on health and beauty hints. A reputable hairstylist can provide answers, too. And, above all, stand tall! Improved posture is equivalent in appearance to a loss of several pounds!

Do you recommend the use of "water pills?"
Diuretics, or "water pills" as they are commonly called, serve very important functions *if prescribed by your doctor.* For example, they may be used to treat high blood pressure. For the healthy person, using water pills to lose weight may result in *temporary* weight reduction. However, as soon as you replace the fluid your body needs, the weight will return. This is normal and essential for good health. *Permanent* weight loss results when body fat is used to provide calories for normal body activities. This is achieved only when you eat fewer calories than you burn up. When insufficient calories are eaten, your body then goes to its fat stores for energy – and you get thinner. Think of this as your stomach growls. This means your body is getting thinner by turning to your body fat for "food."

Is sugar bad for my health?
Most food that the body uses for energy must eventually be converted into glucose, which is a form of sugar, so all sugar cannot be bad. The sugar called glucose comes from other carbohydrate sources such as grains, cereals, fruits, vegetables, sweets or even from proteins. If an excessive percentage of a person's sugar intake comes from sweets such as syrups, honey, soda pop or table sugar, he will be missing important nutrients that would otherwise be

Diet Dialogue

received from grains, cereals, fruits or vegetables. In limited amounts, sugar from sweets in not unsafe for the average person. It adds flavor and variety to the diet and may prevent an extreme craving for sweets that could result in a binge. A few sweet foods are included in *The World's Most Convenient Diet* for these reasons.

If I add vinegar to the diet, will it help dissolve my fat faster?

No! Unfortunately for the dieters of the world, there is no magical food that will dissolve fat. The rumor about vinegar may have gotten started because vinegar and oil (oil is fat) do not mix. Therefore, it was falsely theorized that if vinegar was taken in, fat would come out. Not true. One good thing about vinegar is true, however. You don't have to worry about its caloric content. So add it to salads or fish without worrying.

Do certain foods nourish only certain parts of the body? For example, are carrots good for the eyes and fish good for the brain?

Nutrients travel to the parts of the body where they are needed. It is true that carotene, which can be made into vitamin A, is found in carrots. Vitamin A happens to improve vision in dim light, but is also is important for healthy mucous membranes. The same is true of protein in fish. Protein is needed throughout the entire body for muscles, skin, hair, hormones, enzymes and antibodies!

Will eating only "health food" result in weight loss?

"Health food" is a term that has been used a lot in recent years, but a universal definition is not clear. Assuming by "health food" you mean food found in health food stores, then the answer is no – eating only health foods cannot guarantee weight loss. Honey, black syrup molasses, dried fruits, legumes, wheat germ and other items promoted as health foods are quite high in calories. If the amount eaten is not calculated to match your body's needs, a weight *gain* can actually result.

Can you judge the quality of an egg by the color if its shell?

The color of an eggshell has to do with the breed of chicken that laid the egg. So go ahead and use white, tan, brown or whatever shade chicken egg you prefer.

Is gelatin good for the fingernails?

No. This is a myth that never seems to die. Fingernails do benefit by adequate protein in the diet, but consuming things such as gelatin capsules and powders are not necessary. Actually, the protein in gelatin is of very poor quality. One of the best things you can do for fingernails is wear protective gloves when doing work that might harm them!

Does spot reducing work?

Yes and no. A person's basic body proportions are determined by heredity. For example, some people tend to put on weight in the mid-section while their thighs remain relatively slim. For others, the opposite may be true. In this regard, more dieting will not change your basic proportions. On a positive note, however, a combination of dieting *and* exercise can certainly improve your proportions. Decreasing calories will lessen total body fat. Add to that specific muscle toning exercises, such as for the abdomen, thighs or derriere, and you have the best approach to streamlining your figure.

Is obesity caused by eating too much starch?

Obesity is caused by eating more calories than your body needs for energy. The extra calories are stored as fat, whether they are from carbohydrates (starch), fats, protein (yes – excess protein can make you fat) or alcohol.

Do you recommend the use of weight-reducing machines?

If you mean appropriately designed machines that help you actually work your muscles, these can be helpful in burning calories and toning your physique. If, however, you are talking about devices that merely shake, rub or pound your fat – forget it! *You* have to be doing the work to actually receive the benefit of decreasing your body mass.

What about saunas or special "sweat suits?"

Saunas and clothing designed to make you perspire will only result in *temporary* fluid weight loss that will return as soon as you drink liquids. As we've emphasized already, only the burning of calories in excess of your body's requirements will result in true weight loss.

Chapter Eleven
Thin Conclusions

Thin Conclusions

"This diet was great because it was so easy. Best of all, everyone said to me, 'Wow, have you lost weight!'"

This is the usual reaction of dieters who have successfully used *The World's Most Convenient Diet*. This young woman added: "I do cook some evenings, but it's nice to know there are some very good prepared items I can use and still know I'm not getting too many calories. This diet has made me sit down and eat three meals a day, and that's something I've always said I didn't have time for."

The diet's versatility is often praised by those who have used the plan. They say they like having the lunch options of salads, sandwiches, entrees, soups or yogurt, or even the choice of eating in restaurants. The different breakfasts seem to accommodate many lifestyles. Another often-cited point: the diet offers the chance to sit down with family members and eat what they're having by just following the amounts recommended for home-cooked meals.

Although the diet plan has most often been noted for its simplicity, the quality and quantity of food is another popular aspect. An office worker found she rarely felt hungry with meals she had chosen. "My co-workers wondered how I could eat *Stouffer's®* Glazed Chicken for lunch and still lose weight – but I did. I felt comfortable knowing I didn't have to do a lot of figuring to see if I was doing things the right way. Labels are confusing to me, so I liked only having to check the menus when I made my shopping list."

Once at their goal weight, people have found *The World's Most Convenient Diet* helpful in maintaining it. You will, too. Use the Menu Planner as your guide. The strategy is flexible, but we do have a few suggestions:

Follow the diet three days a week. You might use the menus on weekends and one other day of the week. Maybe a Tuesday, Wednesday and Thursday combination works better for you. On other days of the week, eat sensibly but without following specific menus. You'll probably surprise yourself and find you're accustomed to eating less.

or

Follow the diet for two of three meals each day. Breakfast and lunch combined will yield about 700 calories. The evening meal can be less structured because you've been calorie conscious earlier. If you find yourself "out-to-lunch" fairly often, use the diet for breakfast and dinner instead. This will keep the calorie total for those two meals around 800.

A rule when using any maintenance method: All snack food must come from the Fresh Fruit Stand or Super Salad Bar lists. These are healthy between-meal snacks that are low in calories and high in nutrients. Finally, don't forget to continue your exercise program. The energy expended will be helpful in keeping your weight down – especially on days you've overeaten. Continue to weigh yourself weekly to keep a check on matters.

Whether maintaining your weight after dieting or initially losing it, your secret is having a sincere desire to succeed. This comes with self-motivation. We could list all the health risks of being overweight, but that won't necessarily help motivate people. In diet counseling, forecasting what could happen to your health if a diet isn't followed doesn't always have an impact. If you are feeling symptom-free and healthy at your present weight, it's not threatening to think of consequences down the road.

What *will* work? Make your own personal list of why you will succeed. Your answers may include health reasons, but it's essential the reasons are *your* reasons and not anyone else's. So make that list and update it on a weekly or biweekly basis.

A final word on convenience foods: you may still be surprised to see them included on a weight-loss plan. Don't be. The prepared foods that are part of this diet had to first meet our nutritional criteria. Some products were excluded because of inadequate or excessive amounts of certain nutrients. Calories, sodium, fat, fiber, vitamins and minerals were all considered.

The demand for convenience foods is greater than ever before and will continue to grow. But keeping pace with that consumer demand is a strong trend toward health consciousness. We are excited to see the industry beginning to take steps to meet this demand. The move to prepare food with less fat and calories has enabled many new "light" types of convenience items to be included on this diet. Also evident is the move to prepare more foods with polyunsaturated fats rather than less expensive saturated fats. Lowering the sodium content has been another important factor. Products are now appearing with as much as a one-third reduction in sodium content. Technological advances in both preparation and packaging are resulting in higher-quality products.

After an extensive review of the most recently available nutrient data, we have selected products that can be used on a weight-loss plan when combined wth fresh fruits, vegetables whole grain breads and milk. *The World's Most Convenient Diet* is a simple, sensible and versatile guide to losing weight. Good luck toward your "thin conclusion!"

The Menu-Planner Index

Index to Menu Planner

The following is an alphabetical listing, by food category, of the brand-name products used in *The World's Most Convenient Diet*. For each item, the pages of the menus that include the product are indicated. This list can be used as a handy reference when you are "in the mood" for a certain type of food. For example, how about some pasta tonight??

Bagels
- *Lender's®* Bagels — 52, 53

Bakery Breakfasts — 53

Beans (Also see Soups and Stews)
- *Campbell's®* Beans and Franks — 68
- *Friend's®* Small Pea Baked Beans — 71
- *B & M®* Red Kidney, Small Pea and Yellow Eye Baked Beans — 67, 86

Beef (Also see Pasta and Soups and Stews)
- *Arby's®* French Dip — 61, 83
- *Arby's®* Regular Roast Beef Sandwich — 61, 83
- *Armour Classic Lite™* Beef Pepper Steak — 66
- *Armour Classic Lite™* Turf and Surf — 66, 84
- *Armour Dinner Classic®* Beef Burgundy — 67, 85
- *Armour Dinner Classic®* Beef Stroganoff — 67, 85
- *Armour Dinner Classic®* Sirloin Tips — 85
- *Armour Dinner Classic®* Teriyaki Steak — 85
- *Banquet®* Beef with Gravy Dinner — 86
- *Burger-King®* Hamburger — 61
- *Dairy Queen Brazier®* Single Hamburger — 61
- *Dairy Queen Brazier®* Single Hamburger with Cheese — 83
- *Eckrich® Calorie Watcher™* Slender Sliced Corned Beef — 62, 93
- *Green Giant®* Beef Chow Mein with Rice and Vegetables — 71
- *Green Giant®* Beef Stroganoff with Noodles — 71, 87
- *Green Giant®* Steak and Green Peppers in Sauce with Rice and Vegetables — 72, 88
- *McDonald's®* Cheeseburger — 61

The World's Most Convenient Diet

McDonald's® Quarter Pounder® (no cheese)	83
Pepperidge Farm® Deli, Beef with Barbecue Sauce	72
Pepperidge Farm® Deli, Sliced Beef with Brown Sauce	73
Stouffer's® Lean Cuisine® Oriental Beef in Sauce with Vegetables and Rice	74
Stouffer's® Lean Cuisine® Salisbury Steak with Italian Style Sauce and Vegetables	76, 90
Swanson® Le Menu™ Beef Sirloin Tips	90
Swanson® Le Menu™ Pepper Steak	76, 91
Swanson® Le Menu™ Yankee Pot Roast	76, 91
Taco Bell® Bellbeefer®	61, 83
Taco Bell® Bellbeefer® with Cheese	61
Taco Bell® Tacos	83
Underwood® Roast Beef Spread	65
Van De Kamp's® Beef & Burritos with Chili Salsa	78
Van De Kamp's® Beef Chow Mein Mandarin	91
Van De Kamp's® Beef and Vegetables Szechwan with Rice	78, 91
Van De Kamp's® Shredded Beef Enchiladas	78, 92
Wendy's® Taco Salad	83
Beverages	23
Cereals	
Cold (Ready to Eat)	39
General Mills® Cheerios®	39
General Mills® Corn Total®	39
General Mills® Crispy Wheats 'N Raisins®	39
General Mills® Kix®	39
General Mills® Total®	40
General Mills® Wheaties®	40

The Menu-Planner Index

Kellogg's® All-Bran®	40
Kellogg's® Bran Buds®	40
Kellogg's® Cracklin' Oat Bran™	41
Kellogg's® Crispix®	41
Kellogg's® Frosted Mini-Wheats®	41
Kellogg's® Frosted Krispies™	41
Kellogg's® Fruitful Bran™	42
Kellogg's® Honey and Nut Cornflakes™	42
Kellogg's® Most®	42
Kellogg's® Nutri·Grain®	42
Kellogg's® Product 19®	43
Kellogg's® Raisins, Rice and Rye™	43
Kellogg's® Rice Krispies®	43
Kellogg's® Special K®	43
Nabisco® 100% Bran Cereal	44
Nabisco® Shredded Wheat	44
Nabisco® Spoon Size® Shredded Wheat	44
Nabisco® Team® Flakes Cereal	44
Post® Grape-Nuts® Flakes	45
Post® Fortified Oat Flakes	45
Quaker® Corn Bran	45
Quaker® Cinnamon Life®	45
Quaker® Life®	46
Quaker® Puffed Rice	46
Quaker® Puffed Wheat	46
Quaker® Shredded Wheat	46
Quaker® Bran Chex®	47
Quaker® Corn Chex®	47
Ralston® Crispy Rice®	47
Ralston® Rice Chex®	47
Ralson® Tasteeos®	48
Ralston® Wheat Chex®	48
Ralston® Wheat and Raisin Chex®	48
Hot Cereals	49
Nabisco® Mix 'N Eat Cream of Wheat® Apple 'n Cinnamon	49
Nabisco® Mix 'N Eat Cream of Wheat® Brown Sugar Cinnamon	49

    Nabisco® Mix 'N Eat Cream of Wheat®   **49**
      Honey Graham
    Nabisco® Mix 'N Eat Cream of Wheat®   **50**
      Hot Chocolate
    Nabisco® Mix 'N Eat Cream of Wheat®   **50**
      Maple Brown Sugar
    Nabisco® Mix 'N Eat Cream of Wheat®   **50**
      Original
    Nabisco® Mix 'N Eat Cream of Wheat®   **50**
      Raisins 'n Spice
    Instant Quaker® Oatmeal Apples &   **50**
      Cinnamon
    Instant Quaker® Oatmeal Bran & Raisins **50**
    Instant Quaker® Oatmeal Cinnamon & **50**
      Spice
    Instant Quaker® Oatmeal Honey &   **51**
      Graham
    Instant Quaker® Oatmeal Maple &   **51**
      Brown Sugar
    Instant Quaker® Oatmeal Raisins & Spice **51**
    Instant Quaker® Oatmeal Regular Flavor **51**

Cheese (Also see Pasta)
    Cottage Cheese   **56, 79, 94**
    Green Giant® Macaroni and Cheese   **72**
    Grilled Cheese Sandwich   **94**

Chicken (See Poultry)

Chili (See Soups and Stews)

Cool & Quick Suppers   **93**

Croissants
    Sara Lee Croissant® All Butter Flavor   **55**
    Sara Lee Croissant® Cheese Flavor   **56**
    Sara Lee Croissant® Wheat &   **56**
      Honey Flavor

Crumb Cakes
    Oregon Farms® Blueberry Crumb Cake   **54**
    Oregon Farms® Cheese Crumb Cake   **55**
    Oregon Farms® Cherry Crumb Cake   **55**
    Oregon Farms® French Crumb Cake   **55**

The Menu-Planner Index

Donuts
Hostess® Cinnamon Donut	53
Hostess® Plain Donut	53
Hostess® Powdered Sugar Donut	53
Morton® Donut Shop® Chocolate Iced Donut	54
Morton® Donut Shop® Glazed Donut	54
Morton® Donut Shop® Mini Donut	54
Morton® Mini Honey Bun	54

Eggs   53, 54, 56, 93

Fast Food Fare   61, 83

Fish and Seafood (Also see Pasta, Soups & Stews)

Armour Dinner Classic® Cod Almondine	67, 85
Armour Classic Lite™ Filet of Cod Divan	66, 84
Armour Classic Lite™ Turf and Surf	66, 84
Bumble Bee® Water-Packed Tuna	65, 94
Carnation® The Spreadables® Tuna Salad	62
Chicken of the Sea® Water-Packed Tuna	65, 94
Dining Lite™ Seafood Vegetable Medley	70
Mrs. Paul's® Crispier Crunchier Fish Sticks	72
Mrs. Paul's® Light and Natural Cod Fillets	88
Mrs. Paul's® Light and Natural Flounder Fillets	88
Mrs. Paul's® Light and Natural Sole Fillets	88
Star-Kist® Water-Packed Tuna	65, 94
Stouffer's® Scallops and Shrimp Mariner with Rice	89
Stouffer's® Lean Cuisine® Filet of Fish Divan	75, 90
Stouffer's® Lean Cuisine® Filet of Fish Florentine	75, 90
Wakefield® Filet of Fish with Newburg Sauce	78, 92
Wakefield® Seafood Stuffed Potatoes	78

The World's Most Convenient Diet

Wakefield® Sole with Crab Stuffing and Lemon Sauce	78, 92
Wakefield® Sole Florentine with Mornay Sauce	79, 92

Frankfurters (Also see Beans and Franks)

Armour® Turkey Frank	67

Free Foods 22

French Toast

Aunt Jemima® Cinnamon Swirl French Toast	51
Aunt Jemima® French Toast	51

Fresh Fruit Stand 19

Granola Products

Nature Valley® Granola Bars	56, 65
Nature Valley® Granola Clusters®	57
Nature Valley® Granola and Fruit Bars®	57
Quaker Chewy™ Granola Bar	57, 65

Ham (Also see Beans and Ham and Soups and Stews)

Eckrich® Calorie Watcher™ Chopped Ham	62
Eckrich® Calorie Watcher® Sliced Cooked Ham	63, 93
Eckrich® Calorie Watcher® Sweet Smoked Ham	63
Louis Rich™ Turkey Ham	64
Oscar Mayer® 95% Fat Free Cooked Ham	65
Pepperidge Farm® Deli, Turkey, Ham and Cheese	73

Heat And Eat Suppers 84

Home Cooking Suppers 94

Hot and Hearty Lunches 66

Luncheon Meats (Also see Beef, Poultry, Ham)

Eckrich® Calorie Watcher™ Slender Sliced Pastrami	63
Louis Rich™ Turkey Cotto Salami	63
Louis Rich® Turkey Pastrami	64

The Menu-Planner Index

Oscar Mayer® 90% Fat-Free Bar-B-Q Loaf	64
Oscar Mayer® 93% Fat-Free Canadian Style Bacon	64, 94
Oscar Mayer® 93% Fat-Free Peppered Loaf	65
Macaroni And Cheese (See Cheese)	
Manufacturer's Index	171
Miscellaneous Breakfasts	56
Muffins	
Bays® English Muffin	53
Hostess® Blueberry Muffin	53
Morton® Blueberry Muffin	54
Morton® Corn Muffin	54
Pepperidge Farm® Old Fashioned Blueberry Muffin	55
Pepperidge Farm® Old Fashioned Bran with Raisin Muffin	55
Pepperidge Farm® Old Fashioned Carrot Walnut Muffin	55
Pepperidge Farm® Old Fashioned Cinnamon Swirl Muffin	55
Pepperidge Farm® Old Fashioned Corn Muffin	55
Pepperidge Farm® Old Fashioned Orange-Cranberry Muffin	55
Thomas® English Muffin	53
Wonder® English Muffin	53
Wonder® Raisin Round®	53
Non-Convenience Meals	79, 94
Pasta	
Banquet® Spaghetti with Meat Sauce	67
Dining Lite™ Zucchini Lasagna	70, 87
Franco-American® Beef Ravioli in Meat Sauce	71

Franco-American® Spaghetti with Meatballs in Tomato Sauce	71
Franco-American® Spaghetti in Meat Sauce	71
Green Giant® Lasagna	72, 87
Green Giant® Spaghetti with Meatballs with Tomato Sauce	72
Stouffer's® Cheese Stuffed Pasta Shells with Meat Sauce	73
Stouffer's® Chicken Cacciatore with Spaghetti	73, 88
Stouffer's® Single Serving Lasagna	74, 89
Stouffer's® Linguini with Clam Sauce	74
Stouffer's® Lean Cuisine® Beef and Pork Cannelloni with Mornay Sauce	74, 89
Stouffer's® Lean Cuisine® Cheese Cannelloni with Tomato Sauce	75, 89
Stouffer's® Lean Cuisine® Chicken and Vegetable with Vermicelli	75
Stouffer's® Lean Cuisine® Zucchini Lasagna	76, 90
Van De Kamp's® Creamy Spinach Lasagna	92

Peanut Butter 53

Pizza

La Pizzeria™ Cheese Pizza	72
Stouffer's® Cheese French Bread Pizza	74

Poultry (Also see Pasta and Soup and Stews)
Chicken

Armour Classic Lite™ Chicken Burgundy	66, 84
Armour Classic Lite™ Chicken Oriental	66, 84
Armour Dinner Classic® Chicken Fricassee	67, 85
Banquet® Cookin' Bag Chicken Ala King	67
Dining Lite™ Chickan ala King	70, 86
Dining Lite™ Chicken Aloha	70, 86
Dining Lite™ Chicken Cacciatore	70, 86

The Menu-Planner Index

Dining Lite™ Chicken Vegetable Medley   **70, 87**
Eckrich® Calorie Watcher™ Breast of Chicken   **62**
Green Giant® Chicken Chow Mein with Rice and Vegetables   **71**
Green Giant® Chicken and Broccoli with Rice in Cheese Sauce   **87**
Green Giant® Chicken and Pea Pods in Sauce with Rice and Vegetables   **72, 87**
Kentucky Fried Chicken®   **61**
Stouffer's® Chicken a la King with Rice   **73, 88**
Stouffer's® Chicken Chow Mein without Noodles   **73**
Stouffer's® Lean Cuisine® Chicken Chow Mein with Rice   **75**
Stouffer's® Lean Cuisine® Glazed Chicken with Vegetable Rice   **75, 89**
Swanson® Le Menu™ Chicken a la King   **76, 90**
Swanson® Le Menu™ Breast of Chicken Parmigiana   **91**
Tyson® Chick 'N Quick® Chicken Sticks   **77**
Tyson® Chick 'N Quick® Cordon Bleu Chicken   **77, 91**
Underwood® Chunky Chicken Spread   **65**
Van De Kamp's® Almond Chicken Cantonese with Rice   **92**
Van De Kamp's® Chicken Chow Mein Mandarin   **92**
Van De Kamp's® Chicken Enchilada Suiza   **78**
Weaver® Chicken Au Gratin   **79, 93**
Weaver® Crispy Sticks   **79, 93**
Weaver® Mini-Drums   **79**
Weaver® Rondelets   **79, 93**
Wendy's® Chicken a la King Hot Stuffed Baked Potato   **61**
Wendy's® Chicken Sandwich   **61, 83**
Wendy's® Chicken Sandwich with Cheese   **83**

Turkey
  Armour® Classic Lite™ Turkey Parmesan **66, 84**
  Carnation® The Spreadables® Turkey   62
    Salad
  Eckrich® Calorie Watcher™ Slender   63
    Sliced Smoked Turkey
  Louis Rich™ Oven Roasted Turkey Breast **64, 93**
  Louis Rich® Smoked Turkey Breast   64
  Pepperidge Farm Deli® Turkey, Ham and 73
    Cheese
  Tyson® Turkey Quick® Turkey Pattie   77

Rolls
  King's Hawaiian® Rolls or Bread   53

Salad
  Chef's Salad   79
  Julienne Salad   93
  Super Salad Bar   21

Sample Menu For One Week   29

Seafood (See Fish)

Shopping Guide For The First Week   27

Simple Sandwiches, Etc.   62

Soups and Stews
  Campbell's® Chunky® Old Fashioned   68
    Bean with Ham
  Campbell's® Chunky® Beef Soup   68
  Campbell's® Chunky® Chicken Soup   68
  Campbell's® Chunky® Chili Beef Soup   68, 86
  Campbell's® Chunky® Clam Chowder   69
  Campbell's® Chunky® Mediterranean   69
    Vegetable Soup
  Campbell's® Chunky® Mexicali   69
    Bean Soup
  Campbell's® Chunky® Split Pea with   69
    Ham Soup
  Campbell's® Chunky® Turkey Soup   69
  Campbell's® Chunky® Old Fashioned   69
    Vegetable Beef Soup

The Menu-Planner Index

    Green Giant® Beef Stew   **71, 87**
    Stouffer's® Chili Con Carne with Beans   **77**
    Stouffer's® New England Clam Chowder Soup   **74**
    Stouffer's® Split Pea with Ham Soup   **77, 89**
    Stouffer's® Lean Cuisine® Meatball Stew   **75**
    Tabatchnick's® Bean with Barley Soup   **76**
    Tabatchnick's® Northern Bean Soup   **76**
    Tabatchnick's® Lentil Soup   **77**
    Tabatchnick's® Minestrone Soup   **77**
    Tabatchnick's® Pea Soup   **77**
    Tabatchnick's® Seafood Chowder   **77**
    Wendy's® Chili   **62, 83**

Syrup
    Aunt Jemima® Lite Syrup Product   **51, 52**

Toaster Breakfasts   **51**

Turkey (See Poultry)

Veal
    Armour Classic Lite™ Veal Pepper Steak   **66, 85**

Vitamins With Minerals List   **99**

Waffles
    Aunt Jemima® Jumbo Apple and Cinnamon Waffles   **51**
    Aunt Jemima® Jumbo Blueberry Waffles   **51**
    Aunt Jemima® Jumbo Buttermilk Waffles   **52**
    Aunt Jemima® Jumbo Original Waffles   **52**
    Eggo® Brand Homestyle Waffles Regular   **52**
    Eggo® Brand Homestyle Waffles Apple Cinnamon   **52**
    Eggo® Brand Homestyle Waffles Blueberry   **52**
    Eggo® Brand Homestyle Waffles Buttermilk   **52**
    Eggo® Brand Homestyle Waffles Strawberry   **52**

When You're The Cook: Lunches   **79**

Yogurt
- *Borden's®*   **57, 65**
- *Dannon®*   **57, 65**
- *Meadow Gold®*   **57, 65**
- *Yoplait®*   **57, 65**

Manufacturers' Index

Manufacturers' Index

The following is an alphabetical listing, by manufacturer, of the brand-name products used in *The World's Most Convenient Diet*. For each item, the meals for which the product can be used is indicated. This list can be used as a handy shopping guide for selecting menus that incorporate foods from your favorite companies.

B = Breakfast
L = Lunch
D = Dinner

Arby's®	French Dip	L or D
Arby's®	Regular Roast Beef Sandwich	L or D
Armour Classic Lite™	Beef Pepper Steak	L
Armour Classic Lite™	Chicken Burgundy	L or D
Armour Classic Lite™	Chicken Oriental	L or D
Armour Classic Lite™	Filet of Cod Divan	L or D
Armour Classic Lite™	Turf and Surf	L or D
Armour Classic Lite™	Turkey Parmesan	L or D
Armour Classic Lite™	Veal Pepper Steak	L or D
Armour Dinner Classic®	Beef Burgundy	L or D
Armour Dinner Classic®	Beef Stroganoff	L or D
Armour Dinner Classic®	Chicken Fricassee	L or D
Armour Dinner Classic®	Cod Almondine	L or D
Armour Dinner Classic®	Sirloin Tips	D
Armour Dinner Classic®	Teriyaki Steak	D
Armour®	Turkey Frank	L
Aunt Jemima®	Cinnamon Swirl French Toast	B
Aunt Jemima®	French Toast	B
Aunt Jemima®	Jumbo Apple & Cinnamon Waffles	B
Aunt Jemima®	Jumbo Blueberry Waffles	B
Aunt Jemima®	Jumbo Buttermilk Waffles	B
Aunt Jemima®	Jumbo Original Waffles	B
Aunt Jemima®	Lite Syrup Product	B

B & M®	Red Kidney, Small Pea or Yellow Eye Baked Beans	L or D
Banquet®	Beef with Gravy Dinner	D
Banquet®	Cookin' Bag Chicken Ala King	L
Banquet®	Spaghetti with Meat Sauce	L
Bays®	English Muffin	B
Borden's®	Yogurt – any flavor	B or L
Bumble Bee®	Water-packed Tuna	L or D
Burger King®	Hamburger	L
Campbell's®	Beans and Franks	L
Campbell's®	*Chunky*® Old Fashioned Bean with Ham Soup	L
Campbell's®	*Chunky*® Beef Soup	L
Campbell's®	*Chunky*® Chicken Soup	L
Campbell's®	*Chunky*® Chili Beef Soup	L or D
Campbell's®	*Chunky*® Clam Chowder (Manhattan Style)	L
Campbell's®	*Chunky*® Mediterranean Vegetable Soup	L
Campbell's®	*Chunky*® Mexicali Bean Soup	L
Campbell's®	*Chunky*® Split Pea with Ham Soup	L
Campbell's®	*Chunky*® Turkey Soup	L
Campbell's®	*Chunky*® Old Fashioned Vegetable Beef Soup	L
Carnation®	*The Spreadables*®, Tuna Salad	L
Carnation®	*The Spreadables*®, Turkey Salad	L
Chicken of the Sea®	Water-packed Tuna	L or D

Manufacturers' Index

Dairy Queen Brazier®	Single Hamburger	L
Dairy Queen Brazier®	Single Hamburger with Cheese	D
Dannon®	Yogurt – any flavor	B or L
Dining Lite™	Chicken ala King	L or D
Dining Lite™	Chicken Aloha	L or D
Dining Lite™	Chicken Caccitore	L or D
Dining Lite™	Chicken Vegetable Medley	L or D
Dining Lite™	Seafood Vegetable Medley	L
Dining Lite™	Zucchini Lasagna	L or D
Eckrich® *Calorie Watcher*™	Breast of Chicken	L
Eckrich® *Calorie Watcher*™	Slender Sliced Corned Beef	L or D
Eckrich® *Calorie Watcher*™	Chopped Ham	L
Eckrich® *Calorie Watcher*™	Sliced Cooked Ham	L or D
Eckrich® *Calorie Watcher*™	Sweet Smoked Ham	L
Eckrich® *Calorie Watcher*™	Slender Sliced Pastrami	L
Eckrich® *Calorie Watcher*™	Slender Sliced Smoked Turkey	L
Eggo® *Brand Homestyle Waffles*	Regular	B
Eggo® *Brand Homestyle Waffles*	Apple Cinnamon	B
Eggo® *Brand Homestyle Waffles*	Blueberry	B
Eggo® *Brand Homestyle Waffles*	Buttermilk	B
Eggo® *Brand Homestyle Waffles*	Strawberry	B
Franco-American®	Beef Ravioli in Meat Sauce	L
Franco-American®	Spaghetti with Meatballs in Tomato Sauce	L
Franco-American®	Spaghetti in Meat Sauce	L

Friend's®	Small Pea Baked Beans	L
General Mills®	*Cheerios*®	B
General Mills®	*Corn Total*®	B
General Mills®	*Crispy Wheats 'N Raisins*®	B
General Mills®	*Kix*®	B
General Mills®	*Total*®	B
General Mills®	*Wheaties*®	B
Green Giant®	Beef Chow Mein with Rice and Vegetables	L
Green Giant®	Beef Stew	L or D
Green Giant®	Beef Stroganoff with Noodles	L or D
Green Giant®	Chicken Chow Mein with Rice and Vegetables	L
Green Giant®	Chicken and Broccoli with Rice in Cheese Sauce	D
Green Giant®	Chicken and Pea Pods in Sauce with Rice and Vegetables	L or D
Green Giant®	Lasagna	L or D
Green Giant®	Macaroni and Cheese	L
Green Giant®	Spaghetti with Meatballs with Tomato Sauce	L
Green Giant®	Steak and Green Peppers in Sauce with Rice and Vegetables	L or D
Hostess®	Cinnamon Donut	B
Hostess®	Plain Donut	B
Hostess®	Powdered Sugar Donut	B
Hostess®	Blueberry Muffin	B
Kellogg's®	*All-Bran*®	B
Kellogg's®	*Bran Buds*®	B
Kellogg's®	*Cracklin' Oat Bran*™	B
Kellogg's®	*Crispix*®	B

Manufacturers' Index

Kellogg's®	*Frosted Mini-Wheats®*	B
Kellogg's®	*Frosted Krispies*™	B
Kellogg's®	*Fruitful Bran*™	B
Kellogg's®	*Honey & Nut Cornflakes*™	B
Kellogg's®	*Most®*	B
Kellogg's®	*Nutri-Grain® Corn, Wheat, Wheat & Raisins*	B
Kellogg's®	*Product 19®*	B
Kellogg's®	*Raisins, Rice and Rye*™	B
Kellogg's®	*Rice Krispies®*	B
Kellogg's®	*Special K®*	B
Kentucky Fried Chicken®	Drumstick	L
King's Hawaiian®	Bread	B
King's Hawaiian®	Original Roll	B
La Pizzeria™	Cheese Pizza	L
Lender's®	Bagel, any variety	B
Louis Rich™	Oven Roasted Turkey Breast	L or D
Louis Rich™	Smoked Turkey Breast	L
Louis Rich™	Turkey Cotto Salami	L
Louis Rich™	Turkey Ham	L
Louis Rich™	Turkey Pastrami	L
McDonald's®	Cheeseburger	L
McDonald's®	Quarter Pounder® (no cheese)	D
Meadow Gold®	Yogurt – any flavor	B or L
Morton® Donut Shop®	Chocolate Iced Donut	B
Morton® Donut Shop®	Glazed Donut	B
Morton® Donut Shop®	Mini Donut	B
Morton®	Mini Honey Bun	B
Morton®	Blueberry Muffin	B
Morton®	Corn Muffin	B

Mrs. Paul's®	Crispier Crunchier Fish Sticks	L
Mrs. Paul's®	Light and Natural Cod Fillets	D
Mrs. Paul's®	Light and Natural Flounder Filets	D
Mrs. Paul's®	Light and Natural Sole Fillets	D
Nabisco®	100% Bran Cereal	B
Nabisco®	Shredded Wheat	B
Nabisco®	Spoon Size® Shredded Wheat	B
Nabisco®	Team® Flakes Cereal	B
Nabisco® Mix 'N Eat Cream of Wheat®	Apple 'n Cinnamon	B
Nabisco® Mix 'N Eat Cream of Wheat®	Brown Sugar Cinnamon	B
Nabisco® Mix 'N Eat Cream of Wheat®	Honey Graham	B
Nabisco® Mix 'N Eat Cream of Wheat®	Hot Chocolate	B
Nabisco® Mix 'N Eat Cream of Wheat®	Maple Brown Sugar	B
Nabisco® Mix 'N Eat Cream of Wheat®	Original	B
Nabisco® Mix 'N Eat Cream of Wheat®	Raisins 'n Spice	B
(General Mills®) Nature Valley®	Granola Bar, Almond, Coconut, Cinnamon, Oats 'n Honey, Peanut	B or L
Nature Valley®	Chewy Granola Bar – Apple, Raisin	B or L
Nature Valley®	*Granola Clusters®* Roll	B
Nature Valley®	*Granola & Fruit Bar®* – Apple, Date or Raspberry	B or L

Manufacturers' Index

Oregon Farms®	Blueberry Crumb Cake	B
Oregon Farms®	Cheese Crumb Cake	B
Oregon Farms®	Cherry Crumb Cake	B
Oregon Farms®	French Crumb Cake	B
Oscar Mayer®	90% Fat Free Bar-B-Q Loaf	L
Oscar Mayer®	93% Fat Free Canadian Style Bacon	L or D
Oscar Mayer®	95% Fat Free Cooked Ham	L
Oscar Mayer®	93% Fat Free Peppered Loaf	L
(Campbell's) Pepperidge Farm®	Old Fashioned Blueberry Muffin	B
Pepperidge Farm®	Old Fashioned Bran with Raisin Muffin	B
Pepperidge Farm®	Old Fashioned Carrot Walnut Muffin	B
Pepperidge Farm®	Old Fashioned Cinnamon Swirl Muffin	B
Pepperidge Farm®	Old Fashioned Corn Muffin	B
Pepperidge Farm®	Old Fashioned Orange-Cranberry Muffin	B
Pepperidge Farm® Deli	Beef with Barbecue Sauce	L
Pepperidge Farm® Deli	Sliced Beef with Brown Sauce	L
Pepperidge Farm® Deli	Turkey, Ham and Cheese	L
Post®	*Grape-Nuts*® Flakes	B
Post®	Fortified Oat Flakes	B
Quaker®	Corn Bran	B
Quaker®	*Cinnamon Life*®	B
Quaker®	*Life*®	B
Quaker®	Puffed Rice	B
Quaker®	Puffed Wheat	B

The World's Most Convenient Diet

Quaker®	Shredded Wheat	**B**
Quaker®	Chewy Granola Bars	**B or L**
Instant Quaker® *Oatmeal*	Apples & Cinnamon	**B**
Instant Quaker® *Oatmeal*	Bran & Raisins	**B**
Instant Quaker® *Oatmeal*	Cinnamon & Spice	**B**
Instant Quaker® *Oatmeal*	Honey & Graham	**B**
Instant Quaker® *Oatmeal*	Maple & Brown Sugar	**B**
Instant Quaker® *Oatmeal*	Raisins & Spice	**B**
Instant Quaker® *Oatmeal*	Regular flavor	**B**
Ralston®	*Bran Chex*®	**B**
Ralston®	*Corn Chex*®	**B**
Ralston®	*Crispy Rice*®	**B**
Ralston®	*Rice Chex*®	**B**
Ralston®	*Tasteeos*®	**B**
Ralston®	*Wheat Chex*®	**B**
Ralston®	*Wheat and Raisin Chex*®	**B**
Sara Lee Croissant®	All Butter flavor	**B**
Sara Lee Croissant®	Cheese flavor	**B**
Sara Lee Croissant®	Wheat and Honey	**B**
Star-Kist®	Water-packed Tuna	**L or D**
Stouffer's®	Cheese Stuffed Pasta Shells with Meat Sauce	**L**
Stouffer's®	Chicken a la King with Rice	**L or D**
Stouffer's®	Chicken Cacciatore with Spaghetti	**L or D**
Stouffer's®	Chicken Chow Mein without Noodles	**L**
Stouffer's®	Chili Con Carne with Beans	**L**
Stouffer's®	New England Clam Chowder Soup	**L**
Stouffer's®	Single Serving Lasagna	**L or D**
Stouffer's®	Linguini with Clam Sauce	**L**

Manufacturers' Index

Stouffer's®	Cheese French Bread Pizza	L
Stouffer's®	Scallops & Shrimp Mariner with Rice	D
Stouffer's®	Split Pea with Ham Soup	L or D
Stouffer's® Lean Cuisine®	Beef and Pork Cannelloni with Mornay Sauce	L or D
Stouffer's® Lean Cuisine®	Oriental Beef in Sauce with Vegetables and Rice	L
Stouffer's® Lean Cuisine®	Cheese Cannelloni with Tomato Sauce	L or D
Stouffer's® Lean Cuisine®	Chicken Chow Mein with Rice	L
Stouffer's® Lean Cuisine®	Glazed Chicken with Vegetable Rice	L or D
Stouffer's® Lean Cuisine®	Chicken and Vegetables with Vermicelli	L
Stouffer's® Lean Cuisine®	Filet of Fish Divan	L or D
Stouffer's® Lean Cuisine®	Filet of Fish Florentine	L or D
Stouffer's® Lean Cuisine®	Meatball Stew	L
Stouffer's® Lean Cuisine®	Salisbury Steak with Italian Style Sauce and Vegetables	L or D
Stouffer's® Lean Cuisine®	Zucchini Lasagna	L or D
Swanson® Le Menu™	Beef Sirloin Tips	D
Swanson® Le Menu™	Breast of Chicken Parmigiana	D
Swanson® Le Menu™	Chicken a la King	L or D
Swanson® Le Menu™	Pepper Steak	L or D
Swanson® Le Menu™	Yankee Pot Roast	L or D
Tabatchnick's®	Bean & Barley Soup	L
Tabatchnick's®	Northern Bean Soup	L
Tabatchnick's®	Lentil Soup	L
Tabatchnick's®	Minestrone Soup	L
Tabatchnick's®	Pea Soup	L
Tabatchnick's®	Seafood Chowder	L

Taco Bell®	*Bellbeefer*®	L or D
Taco Bell®	*Bellbeefer*® with Cheese	L
Taco Bell®	Tacos	D
Thomas®	English Muffin	B
Tyson®	*Chick 'N Quick*® Chicken Sticks	L
Tyson®	*Chick 'N Quick*® Cordon Bleu Chicken	L or D
Tyson®	*Turkey Quick*® Turkey Pattie	L
Underwood®	Roast Beef Spread	L
Underwood®	Chunky Chicken Spread	L
Van De Kamp's®	Beef & Bean Burritos with Chili Salsa	L
Van De Kamp's®	Beef Chow Mein Mandarin	D
Van De Kamp's®	Beef and Vegetables Szechwan with Rice	L or D
Van De Kamp's®	Almond Chicken Cantonese with Rice	D
Van De Kamp's®	Chicken Chow Mein Mandarin	D
Van De Kamp's®	Chicken Enchilada Suiza	L
Van De Kamp's®	Creamy Spinach Lasagna	D
Van De Kamp's®	Shredded Beef Enchiladas	L or D
Wakefield®	Filet of Fish with Newburg Sauce	L or D
Wakefield®	Seafood Stuffed Potatoes	L
Wakefield®	Sole with Crab Stuffing and Lemon Sauce	L or D
Wakefield®	Sole Florentine with Mornay Sauce	L or D
Weaver®	Chicken Au Gratin	L or D

Manufacturers' Index

Weaver®	Crispy Sticks	L or D
Weaver®	Mini-Drums, Crispy or Herb 'n Spice Variety	L
Weaver®	Rondelet, Original, Cheese or Italian Variety	L or D
Wendy's®	Chicken á la King Hot Stuffed Baked Potato	L
Wendy's®	Chicken Sandwich	L or D
Wendy's®	Chicken Sandwich with Cheese	D
Wendy's®	Chili	L or D
Wendy's®	Taco Salad	D
Wonder®	English Muffin	B
Wonder®	*Raisin Round®*	B
Yoplait®	*Breakfast Yogurt™* – any flavor	B or L
Yoplait®	Yogurt – any flavor	B or L

References

References

American Drug Index, 28th edition, by Norman F. Billups, Ph.D., R.Ph., Philadelphia, Pa.: J.B. Lippincott Co., 1984.

Controversies in Nutrition edited by Leon Ellenbogen, Ph.D., New York: Churchill Livingstone, Inc. 1981.

The Family Guide to Better Food and Better Health by Ronald Deutsch. New York: Bantam Books, 1979.

Food for Life by F.E. Deatherage, New York and London: Plenum Press, 1975.

Food Science and Nutrition: Current Issues and Answers by Fergus Clydesdale, editor. Englewood Cliffs, N.J.: Prentice Hall Inc., 1979.

Food Science and Technology, 4th edition, by Magnus Pyke. London: John Murray (Publishers) Ltd., 1981.

Food Values of Portions Commonly Used, 13th edition, revised by Jean A.T. Pennington and Helen Nichols Church. Philadelphia: J.B. Lippincott Co., 1980.

Learning to Eat by James M. Ferguson, M.D. Palo Alto, Ca.: Bull Publishing Company, 1975.

Normal and Therapeutic Nutrition, 16th edition, by Corrine Robinson, R.D. and Marilyn Lavler, R.D. New York: MacMillan Publishing Co., 1982.

Nutritive Value of American Foods, Agricultural Handbook No. 456, by Catherine F. Adams. Washington D.C.: U.S. Dept. of Agriculture, 1975.

Recommended Dietary Allowances by the National Research Council. Washington D.C.: National Academy of Sciences, 1980.

Authors' Biographies

After graduating with honors from Kent State University with a Bachelor of Science degree in nutrition, **Linda Lackney** went on to complete a dietetic internship at *University Hospitals of Cleveland* while attending graduate school at Case Western Reserve University. Since receiving her Master of Science degree in nutrition, she has worked for the past several years with kidney patients on hemodialysis.

Ms. Lackney has been active in many professional organizations, including the Cleveland Dietetic Association, Ohio Dietetic Association, Kidney Foundation of Ohio and the Northern and Eastern Ohio Renal Dietitians. In 1983, she received the award for *Recognized Young Dietition of the Year* by the American Dietetic Association. Ms. Lackney has published articles dealing with various aspects of nutrition for kidney patients.

Zoe Ann Komaransky graduated with honors from Ohio State University, earning a Bachelor of Science degree in medical dietetics. During her decade of work as a registered dietitian, her career has focused on nutrition in the health care field. She currently specializes in diet therapy for dialysis patients. In addition, Mrs. Komaransky served as a consultant for patients on weight-loss diets and wrote and conducted a program called, "Weight Loss and the Teenage Girl."

Her professional activities include membership in the American Dietetic Association, Ohio Dietetic Association and Cleveland Dietetic Association.

Working with patients in clinical settings for several years has required Mrs. Komaransky and Ms. Lackney to become knowledgeable in the composition of many brand-name foods so they could achieve as much variety as possible in their clients' special diets. They realized this knowledge could be put to further use by designing a well-balanced weight-loss plan that incorporates brand-name, easy-to-prepare foods.

Thus was born *The World's Most Convenient Diet!*